Yama O. E.
Duru F. I. O.

Chloroquine and body tissues

Funmilayo Akinribido
Yama O. E.
Duru F. I. O.

Chloroquine and body tissues

Reactions of Chloroquine

LAP LAMBERT Academic Publishing

Impressum / Imprint
Bibliografische Information der Deutschen Nationalbibliothek: Die Deutsche
Nationalbibliothek verzeichnet diese Publikation in der Deutschen Nationalbibliografie;
detaillierte bibliografische Daten sind im Internet über http://dnb.d-nb.de abrufbar.
Alle in diesem Buch genannten Marken und Produktnamen unterliegen warenzeichen-,
marken- oder patentrechtlichem Schutz bzw. sind Warenzeichen oder eingetragene
Warenzeichen der jeweiligen Inhaber. Die Wiedergabe von Marken, Produktnamen,
Gebrauchsnamen, Handelsnamen, Warenbezeichnungen u.s.w. in diesem Werk berechtigt
auch ohne besondere Kennzeichnung nicht zu der Annahme, dass solche Namen im Sinne
der Warenzeichen- und Markenschutzgesetzgebung als frei zu betrachten wären und
daher von jedermann benutzt werden dürften.

Bibliographic information published by the Deutsche Nationalbibliothek: The Deutsche
Nationalbibliothek lists this publication in the Deutsche Nationalbibliografie; detailed
bibliographic data are available in the Internet at http://dnb.d-nb.de.
Any brand names and product names mentioned in this book are subject to trademark,
brand or patent protection and are trademarks or registered trademarks of their respective
holders. The use of brand names, product names, common names, trade names, product
descriptions etc. even without a particular marking in this works is in no way to be
construed to mean that such names may be regarded as unrestricted in respect of
trademark and brand protection legislation and could thus be used by anyone.

Coverbild / Cover image: www.ingimage.com

Verlag / Publisher:
LAP LAMBERT Academic Publishing
ist ein Imprint der / is a trademark of
AV Akademikerverlag GmbH & Co. KG
Heinrich-Böcking-Str. 6-8, 66121 Saarbrücken, Deutschland / Germany
Email: info@lap-publishing.com

Herstellung: siehe letzte Seite /
Printed at: see last page
ISBN: 978-3-659-27064-2

DEDICATION

This book is dedicated to Almighty God who gave the insight of the title

ACKNOWLEDGMENT

The International Biomedical &Scientific Research Centre,Ogun State,Nigeria. Acknowledged Akinribido, F.A of the International Biomedical &Scientific Research Centre,Ogun State,Nigeria.Yama, O.E (Dr) of the Department of Anatomy College of Medicine University of Lagos, Idi- Araba, Lagos State, Nigeria.Noronha, C.C(Dr)of the Department of Anatomy College of Medicine University of Lagos, Idi- Araba, Lagos State, Nigeria. Okanlawon, O.A (Professor) of the Department Anatomy College of Medicine University of Lagos, Idi- Araba, Lagos State, Nigeria. Duru, F.I.O(Dr)- of the Department of Anatomy College of Medicine University of Lagos, Idi- Araba, Lagos State, Nigeria, . Mrs. Morenigbade.F and Mrs. Osonbe F.O of Mobid Anatomy Department, College of Medicine, University of Lagos Akoka, Lagos State. For their assistance and support towards the success of this book.

TABLE OF CONTENTS

Chloroquine and Body Tissues

CHAPTER III

TISSUE	CONTROL RATS n=10	CHOLOROQUINE TREATED RATS n=10
Liver (blood vessels)	$4.76 \times 10^{-3} \pm 0.19^a$	$1.93 \times 10\text{-}3 \pm 0.95^b$
Kidney (renal corpuscles)	$4.20 \times 10^{-3} \pm 0.02^a$	$4.15 \times 10\text{-}3 \pm 0.18^b$
Spleen (white pulps)	$5.65 \times 10^{-3} \pm 0.48^a$	$4.0 \times 10\text{-}3 \pm 0.10^b$

a=Mean±S.E.M b=p<0.05

GROUP n=20	MEAN (N/A)
CONTROL (CO)	3.0
TREATED(CQ)	1.0

Chloroquine and Body Tissues

CO =CONTROL CQ =CHLOROQUINE TREATED RATS

TABLE3: MEAN NUMBER OF RENAL CORPUSCLES PER UNIT AREA (N/A)

GROUP n=20	MEAN (N/A)
CONTROL(CO)	2.0
TREATED(CQ)	1.8

CO =CONTROL CQ =CHLOROQUINE TREATED RATS

TABLE 4: MEAN NUMBER OF WHITE PULPS PER UNIT AREA (N/A)

GROUP n=20	MEAN N/A
CONTROL (CO)	1.5
TREATED (CQ)	2.0

CO =CONTROL CQ =CHLOROQUINE TREATED RATS

Chloroquine and Body Tissues

INTRODUCTION

Approximately 50-70% of chloroquine in plasma is bound to plasma proteins. The tissues exhibit particularly high binding to chloroquine especially those containing melanin, for example the retina. Significant binding also occurs in the liver, kidney and spleen. Chloroquine (Resochin, Avloclor, Nivaquine, Arelen) $C_{18}H_{26}CIN_3$ 7- Chloro -4- (4'- diethlyamino-1'-methylamine quinoline). Chloroquine is a white powder with a bitter taste, prepared by chemical synthesis .It is available as sulphate and phosphate salts. The sulphate (1 in 3) and the phosphate (1 in 4) are soluble in water. Chloroquine is best known as an antimalarial agent but it is also used in the treatment of rheumatoid arthritis. Chloroquine is effective against the erythrocytic stages of all four plasmodium species which cause human malaria with the exception of matured plasmodium falciparum gametocytes. The exact mechanisms of the action of chloroquine against malaria parasites are not fully understood. Parasitized red cells accumulate approximately 100-600 times as much chloroquine. The concentration of chloroquine in malaria parasite requires energy and is thought to require a membrane. There are three theories on the way state as that chloroquine, being a basic compound, is protonated in the lysosomes thus raising lysosomal pH. This effect may raise the intralysosomal pH above a critical level all bring about loss lysosomal function. This would reduce the parasite's digestion of heamoglobin, and thus prevent its growth.

Chloroquine intercalates into double stranded DNA and inhibits both DNA and RNA synthesis. The intercalation theory suggests that chloroquine may be bound with increased affinity by certain parts of the genome and be toxic to the malaria parasite by selective accumulation in specific genes, inhibiting their expression. The ferriprotorphyrin IX (FP) which inhibits sequestration of FP into malaria pigment. This could impair heamoglobin degradation and permits damage to the food vacuole sufficient to discharge its Ph gradient.antimalaria activity is possessed equally by the enantiomers of chloroquine and the main metabolite desethlychloroquine is also active against chloroquine- sensitive Plasmodiam.

Chloroquine also has anti- inflammatory activity. The concentrations of chloroquine or hydrochloroquine found in serum in the treatment of rheumatoid disease raise the pH of acid vesicles in mammalian cell within 3-5 min in vitro. This and the observation that the view that chloroquine and hydoxychloroquine act in the rheumatic disease by raising the pH of acid vesicles. Effects of raised vesicle pH include inhibition lysosomal proteolysis, interference with the targeting of acid proteases and inhibition of cellular maturation .raise pH in the macrophage vesicle can interfere with antigen processing. This is thought to be the explanation for the impaired antibody response to pre-exposure to human diploid cell rabies vaccine found in individual receiving concurrent chemoprophyaxis with chloroquine. In addition, chloroquine inhibits the chemotactic response of mononuclear cells and suppresses lymphocytes transformation.

Chloroquine and Body Tissues

It is therefore very important to study the effects of chloroquine on the liver, kidney and spleen.

CHLOROQUINE PHARMACOLOGY

Chloroquine is a medication that is often used to treat or prevent malaria, which is a disease in which parasites infect and attack red blood cells. Although many strains of malaria are resistant to chloroquine, it can still be used as emergency treatment for malaria and several other disorders.

Components

Chloroquine, when taken orally, is typically taken in the form of chloroquine phosphate as a tablet, Drugs.com notes. Chloroquine phosphate tablets come in two dosages: 250 mg and 500 mg, which corresponds to 150 mg and 300 mg of chloroquine, respectively. Chloroquine phosphate tablets also contain inactive ingredients, including colloidal silicon dioxide and microcrystals of cellulose. Other inactive ingredients include either calcium or magnesium stearate and alkali chemicals, which help control the acid-base environment inside the tablets.

Indications

Chloroquine is effective against the asexual forms of the parasites responsible for producing malaria, Infomed explains. It is only effective against the parasite when it is living in red blood cells; consequently, it had no action against parasites that are living in the liver outside of red blood cells. It also is not effective against the gametocytes of the Plasmodium parasites, which are the sexually reproducing forms of the organism. When chloroquine was first discovered it was effective against all strains of the Plasmodium species, but many strains of Plasmodium falciparu--as well as some strains of Plasmodium vivax--have developed resistance to this drug.

Chloroquine can also be used to treat rheumatoid arthritis, lupus, porphyria cutanea tarda, sarcoidosis and liver abscesses caused by amoeba.

Mechanism

The way in which chloroquine is able to treat malaria is not entirely understood. Chloroquine reduces the production of certain enzymes, which can make it difficult for the parasites to survive within red blood cells. Chloroquine also appears to be able to interact with DNA, which could account for some of its anti-parasite activity.

Absorption and Distribution

Chloroquine is rapidly and almost totally absorbed by the gastrointestinal tract, which is why it is typically given orally. Once chloroquine gains access to the blood, approximately 55 percent of it binds to substances in the plasma, Drugs.com explains. Chloroquine is slowly excreted from the body in the urine, though this excretion can be sped up by acidification of the urine. Chloroquine becomes deposited in various tissues; between 200 and 700 times the concentration of the drug in the plasma can be deposited in the liver, lungs, kidneys and spleen. By the time chloroquine is excreted, approximately half of it has been metabolized. The main metabolite of chloroquine is called desethylchloroquine.

Side Effects

Chloroquine can be toxic to the liver and should be used carefully in patients who have a history of liver disease or who consume alcohol or take other potentially hepatotoxic drugs, such as acetaminophen, Medline Plus states. Chloroquine should also be used with care in patients who have hearing problems, as it can cause hearing loss. Patients taking chloroquine need to have their blood tested periodically, as the drug can destroy red blood cells. Patients taking chloroquine may suffer from retinal damage.

CHAPTER I

GROSS ANATOMY OF KIDNEY

ANATOMY OF THE KIDNEYS

Understanding how the urinary system helps maintain homeostasis by removing harmful substances from the blood and regulating water balance in the body is an important part of physiology. Your kidneys, which are the main part of the urinary system, are made up of millions of nephrons that act as individual filtering units and are complex structures themselves. The ureters, urethra, and urinary bladder complete this intricate system.

The urinary system helps maintain homeostasis by regulating water balance and by removing harmful substances from the blood. The blood is filtered by two kidneys, which produce urine, a fluid containing toxic substances and waste products. From each kidney, the urine flows through a tube, the ureter, to the urinary bladder, where it is stored until it is expelled from the body through another tube, the urethra.

The kidneys are surrounded by three layers of tissue:

- The renal fascia is a thin, outer layer of fibrous connective tissue that surrounds each kidney (and the attached adrenal gland) and fastens it to surrounding structures.

Chloroquine and Body Tissues

- The adipose capsule is a middle layer of adipose (fat) tissue that cushions the kidneys.
- The renal capsule is an inner fibrous membrane that prevents the entrance of infections.

Inside the kidney, three major regions are distinguished:

- The renal cortex borders the convex side.
- The renal medulla lies adjacent to the renal cortex. It consists of striated, cone-shaped regions called renal pyramids (medullary pyramids), whose peaks, called renal papillae, face inward. The unstriated regions between the renal pyramids are called renal columns.
- The renal sinus is a cavity that lies adjacent to the renal medulla. The other side of the renal sinus, bordering the concave surface of the kidney, opens to the outside through the renal hilus. The ureter, nerves, and blood and lymphatic vessels enter the kidney on the concave surface through the renal hilus. The renal sinus houses the renal pelvis, a funnel-shaped structure that merges with the ureter.

Blood and nerve supply

Because the major function of the kidneys is to filter the blood, a rich blood supply is delivered by the large renal arteries. The renal artery for each kidney enters the renal hilus and successively branches into segmental arteries and then into interlobar arteries, which pass between the renal pyramids toward the renal cortex. The interlobar arteries then branch into the arcuate arteries, which curve as they pass along the junction of the renal medulla and cortex. Branches of the arcuate arteries, called interlobular arteries, penetrate the renal cortex, where they again branch into afferent arterioles, which enter the filtering mechanisms, or glomeruli, of the nephrons.

The urinary system, (b) the kidney, (c) cortical nephron, and (d) juxtamedullary nephron of the kidneys.

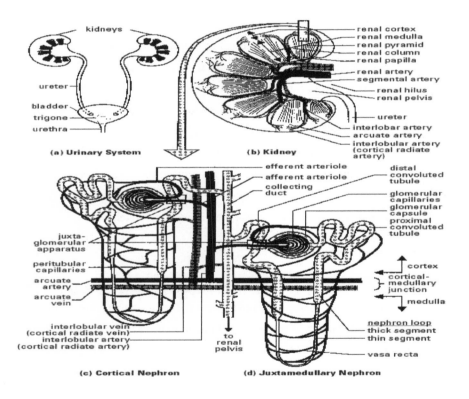

Chloroquine and Body Tissues

Blood leaving the nephrons exits the kidney through veins that trace the same path, in reverse, as the arteries that delivered the blood. Interlobular, arcuate, interlobar, and segmental veins successively merge and exit as a single renal vein.

Autonomic nerves from the renal plexus follow the renal artery into the kidney through the renal hilus. The nerve fibers follow the branching pattern of the renal artery and serve as vasomotor fibers that regulate blood volume. Sympathetic fibers constrict arterioles (decreasing urine output), while less numerous parasympathetic fibers dilate arterioles (increasing urine output).

Nephrons

The kidney consists of over a million individual filtering units called **nephrons**. Each nephron consists of a filtering body, the renal corpuscle, and a urine-collecting and concentrating tube, the renal tubule. The renal corpuscle is an assemblage of two structures, the glomerular capillaries and the glomerular capsule.

- The glomerulus is a dense ball of capillaries (glomerular capillaries) that branches from the afferent arteriole that enters the nephron. Because blood in the glomerular capillaries is under high pressure, substances in the blood that are small enough to pass through the pores (fenestrae, or endothelial fenestrations) in the capillary walls are forced out and into the encircling glomerular capsule. The glomerular capillaries merge, and the remaining blood exits the glomerular capsule through the efferent arteriole.

- The glomerular capsule is a cup-shaped body that encircles the glomerular capillaries and collects the material (filtrate) that is forced out of the glomerular capillaries. The filtrate collects in the interior of the glomerular capsule, the capsular space, which is an area bounded by an inner visceral layer (that faces the glomerular capillaries) and an outer parietal layer. The visceral layer consists of modified simple squamous epithelial cells called podocytes, which project branches that bear fine processes called pedicels. The pedicels' adjacent podocytes mesh to form a dense network that envelops the glomerular capillaries. Spaces between the pedicels, called filtration slits, are openings into the capsular space that allow filtrate to enter the glomerular capsule.

- The renal tubule consists of three sections:
  - The first section, the proximal convoluted tubule (PCT), exits the glomerular capsule as a winding tube in the renal cortex. The wall of the PCT consists of cuboidal cells containing numerous mitochondria and bearing a brush border of dense microvilli that face the lumen (interior cavity). The high-energy yield and large surface area of these cells support their functions of reabsorption and secretion.

Chloroquine and Body Tissues

- The middle of the tubule, the nephron loop, is shaped like a hairpin and consists of a descending limb that drops into the renal medulla and an ascending limb that rises back into the renal cortex. As the loop descends, the tubule suddenly narrows, forming the thin segment of the loop. The loop subsequently widens in the ascending limb, forming the thick segment of the loop. Cells of the nephron loop vary from simple squamous epithelium (descending limb and thin segment of ascending limb) to cuboidal and low columnar epithelium (thick segment of ascending limb) and almost entirely lack microvilli.
- The final section, the distal convoluted tubule (DCT), coils within the renal cortex and empties into the collecting duct. Cells here are cuboidal with few microvilli.

Renal tubules of neighboring nephrons empty urine into a single collecting duct. Here and in the final portions of the DCT, there are cells that respond to the hormones aldosterone and antidiuretic hormone (ADH), and there are cells that secrete H^+ in an effort to maintain proper pH. Various collecting ducts within the medullary pyramids merge to form papillary ducts, which drain eventually into the renal pelvis through the medullary papillae. Urine collects in the renal pelvis and drains out of the kidney through the ureter.

The efferent arteriole carries blood away from the glomerular capillaries to form peritubular capillaries. These capillaries weave around the portions of the renal tubule that lie in the renal cortex. In portions of the nephron loop that descend deep into the renal medulla, the capillaries form loops, called vasa recta, that cross between the ascending and descending limbs. The peritubular capillaries collect water and nutrients from the filtrate in the tubule. They also release substances that are secreted into the tubule to combine with the filtrate in the formation of urine. The capillaries ultimately merge into an interlobular vein, which transports blood away from the nephron region.

There are two kinds of nephrons:

- Cortical nephrons, representing 85 percent of the nephrons in the kidney, have nephron loops that descend only slightly into the renal medulla
- Juxtamedullary nephrons have long nephron loops that descend deep into the renal medulla. Only juxtamedullary nephrons have vasa recta that traverse their nephron loops.

The **juxtaglomerular apparatus (JGA)** is an area of the nephron where the afferent arteriole and the initial portion of the distal convoluted tubule are in close contact. Here, specialized smooth muscle cells of the afferent arteriole, called granular juxtaglomerular (JG) cells, act as mechanoreceptors that monitor blood pressure in the afferent arteriole. In the adjacent distal convoluted tubule, specialized cells, called macula densa, act as chemoreceptors that monitor the concentration of Na^+ and Cl^- in the urine inside the tubule. Together, these cells help regulate blood pressure and the production of urine in the nephron.

Chloroquine and Body Tissues

The operation of the human nephron consists of three processes:

- Glomerular filtration
- Tubular reabsorption
- Tubular secretion

These three processes, which determine the quantity and quality of the urine, are discussed in the following sections.

Glomerular filtration

When blood enters the glomerular capillaries, water and solutes are forced into the glomerular capsule. Passage of cells and certain molecules are restricted as follows:

- The **fenestrae** (pores) of the capillary endothelium are large, permitting all components of blood plasma to pass except blood cells.
- A basement membrane (consisting of extracellular material) that lies between the capillary endothelium and the visceral layer of the glomerular capsule blocks the entrance of large proteins into the glomerular capsule.
- The filtration slits between the pedicels of the podocytes prevent the passage of medium-sized proteins into the glomerular capsule.

The **net filtration pressure (NFP)** determines the quantity of filtrate that is forced into the glomerular capsule. The NFP, estimated at about 10 mm Hg, is the sum of pressures that promote filtration less the sum of those that oppose filtration. The following contribute to the NFP:

- The **glomerular hydrostatic pressure** (blood pressure in the glomerulus) promotes filtration.
- The **glomerular osmotic pressure** inhibits filtration. This pressure is created as a result of the movement of water and solutes out of the glomerular capillaries, while proteins and blood cells remain. This increases the concentration of solutes (thus decreasing the concentration of water) in the glomerular capillaries and therefore promotes the return of water to the glomerular capillaries by osmosis.
- The **capsular hydrostatic pressure** inhibits filtration. This pressure develops as water collects in the glomerular capsule. The more water in the capsule, the greater the pressure.

The **glomerular filtration rate (GFR)** is the rate at which filtrate collectively accumulates in the glomerulus of each nephron. The GFR, about 125 mL/min (180 liters/day), is regulated by the following:

- Renal autoregulation is the ability of the kidney to maintain a constant GFR even when the body's blood pressure fluctuates. Autoregulation is accomplished by cells in the juxtaglomerular apparatus that decrease or increase secretion of a vasoconstrictor substance that dilates or constricts, respectively, the afferent arteriole.
- Neural regulation of GFR occurs when vasoconstrictor fibers of the sympathetic nervous system constrict afferent arterioles. Such

Chloroquine and Body Tissues

stimulation may occur during exercise, stress, or other fight-or-flight conditions and results in a decrease in urine production.

- Hormonal control of GFR is accomplished by the renin/angiotensinogen mechanism. When cells of the juxtaglomerular apparatus detect a decrease in blood pressure in the afferent arteriole or a decrease in solute (Na^+ and Cl^-) concentrations in the distal tubule, they secrete the enzyme renin. Renin converts angiotensinogen (a plasma protein produced by the liver) to angiotensin I. Angiotensin I in turn is converted to angiotensin II by the angiotensin-converting enzyme (ACE), an enzyme produced principally by capillary endothelium in the lungs. Angiotensin II circulates in the blood and increases GFR by doing the following:
  - Constricting blood vessels throughout the body, causing the blood pressure to rise
  - Stimulating the adrenal cortex to secrete aldosterone, a hormone that increases blood pressure by decreasing water output by the kidneys

Tubular reabsorption

In healthy kidneys, nearly all of the desirable organic substances (proteins, amino acids, glucose) are reabsorbed by the cells that line the renal tube. These substances then move into the peritubular capillaries that surround the tubule. Most of the water (usually more than 99 percent of it) and many ions are reabsorbed as well, but the amounts are regulated so that blood volume,

Chloroquine and Body Tissues

pressure, and ion concentration are maintained within required levels for homeostasis.

Reabsorbed substances move from the lumen of the renal tubule to the lumen of a peritubular capillary. Three membranes are traversed:

- The luminal membrane, or the side of the tubule cells facing the tubule lumen
- The basolateral membrane, or the side of the tubule cells facing the interstitial fluids
- The endothelium of the capillaries

Tight junctions between tubule cells prevent substances from leaking out between the cells. Movement of substances out of the tubule, then, must occur through the cells, either by active transport (requiring ATP) or by passive transport processes. Once outside of the tubule and in the interstitial fluids, substances move into the peritubular capillaries or vasa recta by passive processes. The reabsorption of most substances from the tubule to the interstitial fluids requires a membrane-bound transport protein that carries these substances across the tubule cell membrane by active transport. When all of the available transport proteins are being used, the rate of reabsorption reaches a transport maximum (Tm), and substances that cannot be transported are lost in the urine.

The following mechanisms direct tubular reabsorption in the indicated regions:

Chloroquine and Body Tissues

- *Active transport of Na^+ (in the PCT, DCT, and collecting duct).* Because Na^+ concentration is low inside tubular cells, Na^+ enters the tubular cells (across the luminal membrane) by passive diffusion. At the other side of the tubule cells, the basolateral membrane bears proteins that function as sodium-potassium (Na^+-K^+) pumps. These pumps use ATP to simultaneously export Na^+ while importing K^+. Thus, Na^+ in the tubule cells is transported out of the cells and into the interstitial fluid by active transport. The Na^+ in the interstitial fluid then enters the capillaries by passive diffusion. (The K^+ that is transported into the cell leaks back passively into the interstitial fluid.)

- *Symporter transport (secondary active transport) of nutrients and ions (in the PCT and nephron loop).* Various nutrients, such as glucose and amino acids, and certain ions (K^+ and Cl^-) in the thick ascending limb of the nephron loop are transported into the tubule cells by the action of Na^+ symporters. A Na^+ symporter is a transport protein that carries both Na^+ and another molecule, such as glucose, across a membrane in the same direction. Movement of glucose and other nutrients from the tubular lumen into the tubule cells occurs in this fashion. The process requires a low concentration of Na^+ inside the cells, a condition maintained by the Na^+-K^+ pump operating on the basolateral membranes of the tubule cells. The movement of nutrients into cells by this mechanism is referred to as secondary active transport, because the ATP-requiring mechanism is the Na^+-K^+ pump and not the symporter itself. Once inside the tubular cells, nutrients move into the interstitial fluid and into the capillaries by passive processes.

- *Passive transport of H_2O by osmosis (in the PCT and DCT).* The buildup of Na^+ in the peritubular capillaries creates a concentration gradient across which water passively moves, from tubule to capillaries, by osmosis. Thus, the reabsorption of Na^+ by active transport generates the subsequent reabsorption of H_2O by passive transport, a process called obligatory H_2O reabsorption.

- *Passive transport of various solutes by diffusion (in the PCT and DCT, and collecting duct).* As H_2O moves from the tubule to the capillaries, various solutes such as K^+, Cl^-, HCO_3^-, and urea become more concentrated in the tubule. As a result, these solutes follow the water, moving by diffusion out of the tubule and into capillaries where their concentrations are lower, a process called solvent drag. Also, the accumulation of the positively charged Na^+ in the capillaries creates an electrical gradient that attracts (by diffusion) negatively charged ions (Cl^-, HCO_3^-).

- *H_2O and solute transport regulated by hormones (in the DCT and collecting duct).* The permeability of the DCT and collecting duct and the resultant reabsorption of H_2O and Na^+ are controlled by two hormones:
  - Aldosterone increases the reabsorption of Na^+ and H_2O by stimulating an increase in the number of Na^+-K^+ pump proteins in the principal cells that line the DCT and collecting duct.

Chloroquine and Body Tissues

o Antidiuretic hormone (ADH) increases H_2O reabsorption by stimulating an increase in the number of H_2O-channel proteins in the principal cells of the collecting duct.

Tubular secretion

In contrast to tubular reabsorption, which returns substances to the blood, tubular secretion removes substances from the blood and secretes them into the filtrate. Secreted substances include H^+, K^+, NH_4^+ (ammonium ion), creatinine (a waste product of muscle contraction), and various other substances (including penicillin and other drugs). Secretion occurs in portions of the PCT, DCT, and collecting duct.

- *Secretion of H^+*. Because a decrease in H^+ causes a rise in pH (a decrease in acidity), H^+ secretion into the renal tubule is a mechanism for raising blood pH. Various acids produced by cellular metabolism accumulate in the blood and require that their presence be neutralized by removing H^+. In addition, CO_2, also a metabolic byproduct, combines with water (catalyzed by the enzyme carbonic anhydrase) to produce carbonic acid (H_2CO_3), which dissociates to produce H^+, as follows:

$$CO_2 + H_2O \longleftrightarrow H_2CO_3 \longleftrightarrow H^+ + HCO_3^-$$

This chemical reaction occurs in either direction (it is reversible) depending on the concentration of the various reactants. As a result, if

HCO_3^- increases in the blood, it acts as a buffer of H^+, combining with it (and effectively removing it) to produce CO_2 and H_2O. CO_2 in tubular cells of the collecting duct combines with H_2O to form H^+ and HCO_3^-. The CO_2 may originate in the tubular cells or it may enter these cells by diffusion from the renal tubule, interstitial fluids, or peritubular capillaries. In the tubule cell, Na^+/H^+ antiporters, enzymes that move transported substances in opposite directions, transport H^+ across the luminal membrane into the tubule while importing Na^+. Inside the tubule, H^+ may combine with any of several buffers that entered the tubule as filtrate (HCO_3^-, NH_3, or HPO_4^{2-}). If HCO_3^- is the buffer, then H_2CO_3 is formed, producing H_2O and CO_2. The CO_2 then enters the tubular cell, where it can combine with H_2O again. If H^+ combines with another buffer, it is excreted in the urine. Regardless of the fate of the H+ in the tubule, the HCO_3^- produced in the first step is transported across the basolateral membrane by an HCO_3^-/Cl^- antiporter. The HCO_3^- enters the peritubular capillaries, where it combines with the H^+ in the blood and increases the blood pH. Note that the blood pH is increased by adding HCO_3^- to the blood, not by removing H^+.

Secretion of NH_3. When amino acids are broken down, they produce toxic NH_3. The liver converts most NH_3 to urea, a less toxic substance. Both enter the filtrate during glomerular filtration and are excreted in the urine. However, when the blood is very acidic, the tubule cells break down the amino acid glutamate, producing NH_3 and HCO_3^-. The NH_3 combines with H^+, forming NH_4^+, which is transported across the luminal membrane by a Na^+ antiporter and excreted in the urine. The HCO_3^- moves to the blood (as discussed earlier for H^+ secretion) and increases blood pH.

- *Secretion of K^+*. Nearly all of the K^+ in filtrate is reabsorbed during tubular reabsorption. When reabsorbed quantities exceed body requirements, excess K^+ is secreted back into the filtrate in the collecting duct and final regions of the DCT. Because aldosterone stimulates an increase in Na^+/K^+ pumps, K^+ secretion (as well as Na^+ reabsorption) increases with aldosterone.

GROSS ANATOMY OF LIVER

Liver

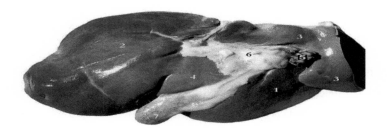

Chloroquine and Body Tissues

Liver of a sheep: (1) right lobe, (2) left lobe, (3) caudate lobe, (4) quadrate lobe, (5) hepatic artery and portal vein, (6) hepatic lymph nodes, (7) gall bladder

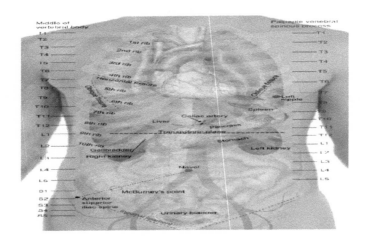

Surface projections of the organs of the trunk, showing liver in center

The **liver** is a vital organ present in vertebrates and some other animals. It has a wide range of functions, including detoxification, protein synthesis, and production of biochemicals necessary for digestion. The liver is necessary for survival; there is currently no way to compensate for the absence of liver function long term, although liver dialysis can be used short term.

Chloroquine and Body Tissues

This organ plays a major role in metabolism and has a number of functions in the body, including glycogen storage, decomposition of red blood cells, plasma protein synthesis, hormone production, and detoxification. It lies below the diaphragm in the abdominal-pelvic region of the abdomen. It produces bile, an alkaline compound which aids in digestion via the emulsification of lipids. The liver's highly specialized tissues regulate a wide variety of high-volume biochemical reactions, including the synthesis and breakdown of small and complex molecules, many of which are necessary for normal vital functions.

Medical terms related to the liver often start in *hepato-* or *hepatic* from the Greek word for liver, *hēpar* (παρ   ).

Anatomy

The liver is a reddish brown organ with four lobes of unequal size and shape. A human liver normally weighs 1.44–1.66 kg (3.2–3.7 lb), and is a soft, pinkish-brown, triangular organ. It is both the largest internal organ (the skin being the largest organ overall) and the largest gland in the human body. It is located in the right upper quadrant of the abdominal cavity, resting just below the diaphragm. The liver lies to the right of the stomach and overlies the gallbladder. It is connected to two large blood vessels, one called the hepatic artery and one called the portal vein. The hepatic artery carries blood from the aorta, whereas the portal vein carries blood containing digested nutrients from the entire gastrointestinal tract and also from the spleen and pancreas. These

Chloroquine and Body Tissues

blood vessels subdivide into capillaries, which then lead to a lobule. Each lobule is made up of millions of hepatic cells which are the basic metabolic cells. Lobules are the functional units of the liver.

Cell types

Two major types of cells populate the liver lobes: parenchymal and non-parenchymal cells. 80% of the liver volume is occupied by parenchymal cells commonly referred to as hepatocytes. Non-parenchymal cells constitute 40% of the total number of liver cells but only 6.5% of its volume. Sinusoidal endothelial cells, kupffer cells and hepatic stellate cells are some of the non-parenchymal cells that line the hepatic sinusoid.

Blood flow

The liver gets a dual blood supply from the hepatic portal vein and hepatic arteries. Supplying approximately 75% of the liver's blood supply, the hepatic portal vein carries venous blood drained from the spleen, gastrointestinal tract, and its associated organs. The hepatic arteries supply arterial blood to the liver, accounting for the remainder of its blood flow. Oxygen is provided from both sources; approximately half of the liver's oxygen demand is met by the hepatic portal vein, and half is met by the hepatic arteries.
Blood flows through the liver sinusoids and empties into the central vein of each lobule. The central veins coalesce into hepatic veins, which leave the liver.

Biliary flow

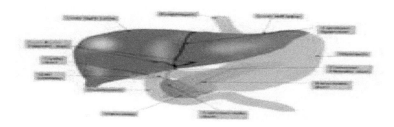

The biliary tree

The term *biliary tree* is derived from the arboreal branches of the bile ducts. The bile produced in the liver is collected in bile canaliculi, which merge to form bile ducts. Within the liver, these ducts are called *intrahepatic* (within the liver) bile ducts, and once they exit the liver they are considered *extrahepatic* (outside the liver). The intrahepatic ducts eventually drain into the right and left hepatic ducts, which merge to form the common hepatic duct. The cystic duct from the gallbladder joins with the common hepatic duct to form the common bile duct.

Bile can either drain directly into the duodenum via the common bile duct, or be temporarily stored in the gallbladder via the cystic duct. The common bile duct and the pancreatic duct enter the second part of the duodenum together at the ampulla of Vater.

Surface anatomy

Peritoneal ligaments

Apart from a patch where it connects to the diaphragm (the so-called "bare area"), the liver is covered entirely by visceral peritoneum, a thin, double-layered membrane that reduces friction against other organs. The peritoneum folds back on itself to form the falciform ligament and the right and left triangular ligaments.

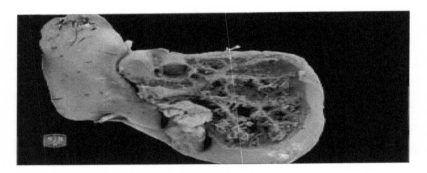

Dissection of portal vein in right lobe of liver

These "lits" are in no way related to the true anatomic ligaments in joints, and have essentially no known functional importance, but they are easily recognizable surface landmarks. An exception to this is the falciform ligament, which attaches the liver to the posterior portion of the anterior body wall.

Lobes

Traditional gross anatomy divided the liver into four lobes based on surface features. The falciform ligament is visible on the front (anterior side) of the liver. This divides the liver into a left anatomical lobe, and a right anatomical lobe. If the liver is flipped over, to look at it from behind (the visceral surface), there are two additional lobes between the right and left. These are the caudate lobe (the more superior) and the quadrate lobe (the more inferior).

From behind, the lobes are divided up by the ligamentum venosum and ligamentum teres (anything left of these is the left lobe). The transverse fissure (or *porta hepatis*) divides the caudate from the quadrate lobe, and the right sagittal fossa, which the inferior vena cava runs over, separates these two lobes from the right lobe.

Each of the lobes is made up of lobules; a vein goes from the centre, which then joins to the hepatic vein to carry blood out from the liver.

On the surface of the lobules, there are ducts, veins and arteries that carry fluids to and from them.

Functional anatomy

Correspondence between anatomic lobes and Couinaud segments

Segment*	Couinaud segments
Caudate	1
Lateral	2, 3
Medial	4a, 4b
Right	5, 6, 7, 8

* or lobe, in the case of the caudate lobe

Each number in the list corresponds to one in the table.

1. Caudate

2. Superior subsegment of the lateral segment

3. Inferior subsegment of the lateral segment

4a. Superior subsegment of the medial segment

4b. Inferior subsegment of the medial segment

5. Inferior subsegment of the anterior segment

6. Inferior subsegment of the posterior segment

7. Superior subsegment of the posterior segment

8. Superior subsegment of the anterior segment

The central area where the common bile duct, hepatic portal vein, and hepatic artery proper enter is the hilum or "porta hepatis". The duct, vein, and artery divide into left and right branches, and the portions of the liver supplied by these branches constitute the functional left and right lobes.

The functional lobes are separated by an imaginary plane joining the gallbladder fossa to the inferior vena cava. The plane separates the liver into the true right and left lobes. The middle hepatic vein also demarcates the true right and left lobes. The right lobe is further divided into an anterior and posterior segment by the right hepatic vein. The left lobe is divided into the medial and lateral segments by the left hepatic vein. The fissure for the ligamentum teres also separates the medial and lateral segments. The medial segment is also called the quadrate lobe. In the widely used Couinaud (or "French") system, the functional lobes are further divided into a total of eight subsegments based on a transverse plane through the bifurcation of the main portal vein. The caudate lobe is a separate structure which receives blood flow from both the right- and left-sided vascular branches.

In other animals

The liver is found in all vertebrates, and is typically the largest visceral organ. Its form varies considerably in different species, and is largely determined by the shape and arrangement of the surrounding organs. Nonetheless, in most species it is divided into right and left lobes; exceptions to this general rule include snakes, where the shape of the body necessitates a simple cigar-like form. The internal structure of the liver is broadly similar in all vertebrates.

Chloroquine and Body Tissues

An organ sometimes referred to as a liver is found associated with the digestive tract of the primitive chordate *Amphioxus*. However, this is an enzyme secreting gland, not a metabolic organ, and it is unclear how truly homologous it is to the vertebrate liver.

Physiology

The various functions of the liver are carried out by the liver cells or hepatocytes. Currently, there is no artificial organ or device capable of emulating all the functions of the liver. Some functions can be emulated by liver dialysis, an experimental treatment for liver failure. The liver is thought to be responsible for up to 500 separate functions, usually in combination with other systems and organs.

Synthesis

Further information: Proteins produced and secreted by the liver

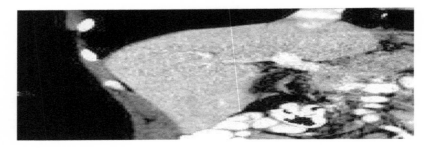

Chloroquine and Body Tissues

A CT scan in which the liver and portal vein are shown.

- A large part of amino acid synthesis
- The liver performs several roles in carbohydrate metabolism:
  - *Gluconeogenesis* (the synthesis of glucose from certain amino acids, lactate or glycerol)
  - *Glycogenolysis* (the breakdown of glycogen into glucose)
  - *Glycogenesis* (the formation of glycogen from glucose)(muscle tissues can also do this)
- The liver is responsible for the mainstay of protein metabolism, synthesis as well as degradation.
- The liver also performs several roles in lipid metabolism:
  - *Cholesterol synthesis*
  - *Lipogenesis*, the production of triglycerides (fats).
  - A bulk of the lipoproteins are synthesized in the liver.
- The liver produces coagulation factors I (fibrinogen), II (prothrombin), V, VII, IX, X and XI, as well as protein C, protein S and antithrombin.
- In the first trimester fetus, the liver is the main site of red blood cell production. By the 32nd week of gestation, the bone marrow has almost completely taken over that task.
- The liver produces and excretes bile (a yellowish liquid) required for emulsifying fats. Some of the bile drains directly into the duodenum, and some is stored in the gallbladder.

- The liver also produces insulin-like growth factor 1 (IGF-1), a polypeptide protein hormone that plays an important role in childhood growth and continues to have anabolic effects in adults.
- The liver is a major site of thrombopoietin production. Thrombopoietin is a glycoprotein hormone that regulates the production of platelets by the bone marrow.

Breakdown

- The breakdown of insulin and other hormones
- The liver glucoronidates bilirubin, facilitating its excretion into bile.
- The liver breaks down or modifies toxic substances (e.g., methylation) and most medicinal products in a process called drug metabolism. This sometimes results in toxication, when the metabolite is more toxic than its precursor. Preferably, the toxins are conjugated to avail excretion in bile or urine.
- The liver converts ammonia to urea (urea cycle).

Other functions

- The liver stores a multitude of substances, including glucose (in the form of glycogen), vitamin A (1–2 years' supply), vitamin D (1–4 months' supply), vitamin B12 (1–3 years' supply), iron, and copper.
- The liver is responsible for immunological effects—the reticuloendothelial system of the liver contains many immunologically

active cells, acting as a 'sieve' for antigens carried to it via the portal system.

- The liver produces albumin, the major osmolar component of blood serum.
- The liver synthesizes angiotensinogen, a hormone that is responsible for raising the blood pressure when activated by renin, an enzyme that is released when the kidney senses low blood pressure.

Relation to medicine and pharmacology

The oxidative capacity of the liver decreases with aging and therefore, benzodiazepines (BZDs) that require oxidation are more likely to accumulate to toxic levels. Therefore, those with shorter half-lives, such as lorazepam and oxazepam are preferred when benzodiazepines are required in regards to geriatric medicine.

Diseases of the liver

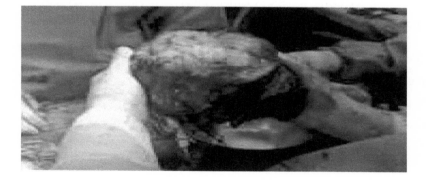

Chloroquine and Body Tissues

Left lobe liver tumor

The liver supports almost every organ in the body and is vital for survival. Because of its strategic location and multidimensional functions, the liver is also prone to many diseases.

The most common include: Infections such as hepatitis A, B, C, D, E, alcohol damage, fatty liver, cirrhosis, cancer, drug damage (particularly by acetaminophen (paracetamol) and cancer drugs).

Many diseases of the liver are accompanied by jaundice caused by increased levels of bilirubin in the system. The bilirubin results from the breakup of the hemoglobin of dead red blood cells; normally, the liver removes bilirubin from the blood and excretes it through bile.

There are also many pediatric liver diseases including biliary atresia, alpha-1 antitrypsin deficiency, alagille syndrome, progressive familial intrahepatic cholestasis, and Langerhans cell histiocytosis, to name but a few.

Diseases that interfere with liver function will lead to derangement of these processes. However, the liver has a great capacity to regenerate and has a large reserve capacity. In most cases, the liver only produces symptoms after extensive damage.

Liver diseases may be diagnosed by liver function tests, for example, by production of acute phase proteins.

Disease symptoms

The classic symptoms of liver damage include the following:

- **Pale stools** occur when stercobilin, a brown pigment, is absent from the stool. Stercobilin is derived from bilirubin metabolites produced in the liver.
- **Dark urine** occurs when bilirubin mixes with urine
- **Jaundice** (yellow skin and/or whites of the eyes) This is where bilirubin deposits in skin, causing an intense itch. Itching is the most common complaint by people who have liver failure. Often this itch cannot be relieved by drugs.
- **Swelling** of the abdomen, ankles and feet occurs because the liver fails to make albumin.
- **Excessive fatigue** occurs from a generalized loss of nutrients, minerals and vitamins.
- **Bruising** and easy bleeding are other features of liver disease. The liver makes substances which help prevent bleeding. When liver damage occurs, these substances are no longer present and severe bleeding can occur.

Diagnosis

The diagnosis of liver function is made by blood tests. Liver function tests can readily pinpoint the extent of liver damage. If infection is suspected, then other serological tests are done. Sometimes, one may require an ultrasound or a CT scan to produce an image of the liver.

Physical examination of the liver is not accurate in determining the extent of liver damage. It can only reveal presence of tenderness or the size of liver, but in all cases, some type of radiological study is required to examine it.

Biopsy / scan

Damage to the liver is sometimes determined with a biopsy, particularly when the cause of liver damage is unknown. In the 21st century they were largely replaced by high-resolution radiographic scans. The latter do not require ultrasound guidance, lab involvement, microscopic analysis, organ damage, pain, or patient sedation; and the results are available immediately on a computer screen.

In a biopsy, a needle is inserted into the skin just below the rib cage and a tissue sample obtained. The tissue is sent to the laboratory, where it is analyzed under a microscope. Sometimes, a radiologist may assist the physician performing a liver biopsy by providing ultrasound guidance.

Regeneration

The liver is the only internal human organ capable of natural regeneration of lost tissue; as little as 25% of a liver can regenerate into a whole liver. This is, however, not true regeneration but rather compensatory growth. The lobes that are removed do not regrow and the growth of the liver is a restoration of function, not original form. This contrasts with true regeneration where both original function and form are restored.

This is predominantly due to the hepatocytes re-entering the cell cycle. That is, the hepatocytes go from the quiescent G0 phase to the G1 phase and undergo mitosis. This process is activated by the p75 receptors. There is also some evidence of bipotential stem cells, called hepatic oval cells or ovalocytes (not to be confused with oval red blood cells of ovalocytosis), which are thought to reside in the canals of Hering. These cells can differentiate into either hepatocytes or cholangiocytes, the latter being the cells that line the bile ducts.

Scientific and medical works about liver regeneration often refer to the Greek Titan Prometheus who was chained to a rock in the Caucasus where, each day, his liver was devoured by an eagle, only to grow back each night. Some think the myth indicates the ancient Greeks knew about the liver's remarkable capacity for self-repair, though this claim has been challenged.

Liver transplantation

Human liver transplants were first performed by Thomas Starzl in the United States and Roy Calne in Cambridge, England in 1963 and 1965, respectively.

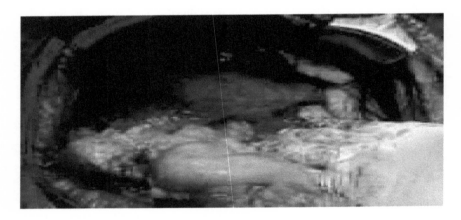

After resection of left lobe liver tumor

Liver transplantation is the only option for those with irreversible liver failure. Most transplants are done for chronic liver diseases leading to cirrhosis, such as chronic hepatitis C, alcoholism, autoimmune hepatitis, and many others. Less commonly, liver transplantation is done for fulminant hepatic failure, in which liver failure occurs over days to weeks.

Liver allografts for transplant usually come from donors who have died from fatal brain injury. Living donor liver transplantation is a technique in which a portion of a living person's liver is removed and used to replace the entire liver of the recipient. This was first performed in 1989 for pediatric liver transplantation. Only 20 percent of an adult's liver (Couinaud segments 2 and 3) is needed to serve as a liver allograft for an infant or small child.

More recently, adult-to-adult liver transplantation has been done using the donor's right hepatic lobe, which amounts to 60 percent of the liver. Due to the ability of the liver to regenerate, both the donor and recipient end up with normal liver function if all goes well. This procedure is more controversial, as it entails performing a much larger operation on the donor, and indeed there have been at least two donor deaths out of the first several hundred cases. A recent publication has addressed the problem of donor mortality, and at least 14 cases have been found. The risk of postoperative complications (and death) is far greater in right-sided operations than that in left-sided operations.

With the recent advances of noninvasive imaging, living liver donors usually have to undergo imaging examinations for liver anatomy to decide if the anatomy is feasible for donation. The evaluation is usually performed by multidetector row computed tomography (MDCT) and magnetic resonance imaging (MRI). MDCT is good in vascular anatomy and volumetry. MRI is used for biliary tree anatomy. Donors with very unusual vascular anatomy, which makes them unsuitable for donation, could be screened out to avoid unnecessary operations.

Chloroquine and Body Tissues

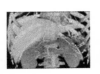

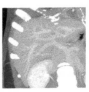

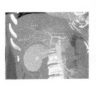 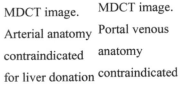 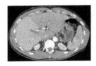

MDCT image. Arterial anatomy contraindicated for liver donation

MDCT image. Portal venous anatomy contraindicated for liver donation

MDCT image. 3D image created by MDCT can clearly visualize the liver, measure the liver volume, and plan the dissection plane to facilitate the liver transplantation procedure.

Phase contrast CT image. Contrast is perfusing the right liver but not the left due to a left portal vein thrombus.

Development

Organogenesis

The origins of the liver lie in both the ventral portion of the foregut endoderm (endoderm being one of the 3 embryonic germ cell layers) and the constituents of the adjacent septum transversum mesenchyme. In human embryo, the hepatic diverticulum is the tube of endoderm that extends out from the foregut into the surrounding mesenchyme. The mesenchyme of septum transversum induces this endoderm to proliferate, to branch, and to form the glandular epithelium of the liver. A portion of the hepatic diverticulum (that region closest to the digestive tube) continues to function as the drainage duct of the liver, and a branch from this duct produces the gallbladder Besides of signals from the septum transversum mesenchyme, fibroblast growth factor from the developing heart also contribute to hepatic competence, along with retinoic acid emanating from the lateral plate mesoderm. The hepatic endodermal cells undergo a morphological transition from columnar to pseudostratified resulting in thickening into the early liver bud. Their expansion forms a population of the bipotential hepatoblasts. Hepatic stellate cells are derived from mesenchyme.

After migration of hepatoblasts into the septum transversum mesenchyme, the hepatic architecture begins to be established, with sinusoids and bile canaliculi appearing. The liver bud separates into the lobes. The left umbilical vein becomes the ductus venosus and the right vitelline vein becomes the portal vein. The expanding liver bud is colonized by hematopoietic cells. The bipotential hepatoblasts begin differentiating into biliary epithelial cells and hepatocytes. The biliary epithelial cells differentiate from hepatoblasts around portal veins, first producing a monolayer, and then a bilayer of cuboidal cells. In ductal plate, focal dilations emerge at points in the bilayer, become surrounded by portal mesenchyme, and undergo tubulogenesis into intrahepatic bile ducts. Hepatoblasts not adjacent to portal veins instead differentiate into hepatocytes and arrange into cords lined by sinudoidal epithelial cells and bile canaliculi. Once hepatoblasts are specified into

Chloroquine and Body Tissues

hepatocytes and undergo further expansion, they begin acquiring the functions of a mature hepatocyte, and eventually mature hepatocytes appear as highly polarized epithelial cells with abundant glycogen accumulation. In the adult liver, hepatocytes are not equivalent, with position along the portocentrovenular axis within a liver lobule dictating expression of metabolic genes involved in drug metabolism, carbohydrate metabolism, ammonia detoxification, and bile production and secretion. WNT/β-catenin has now been identified to be playing a key role in this phenomenon.

Fetal blood supply

In the growing fetus, a major source of blood to the liver is the umbilical vein which supplies nutrients to the growing fetus. The umbilical vein enters the abdomen at the umbilicus, and passes upward along the free margin of the falciform ligament of the liver to the inferior surface of the liver. There it joins with the left branch of the portal vein. The ductus venosus carries blood from the left portal vein to the left hepatic vein and then to the inferior vena cava, allowing placental blood to bypass the liver.

In the fetus, the liver develops throughout normal gestation, and does not perform the normal filtration of the infant liver. The liver does not perform digestive processes because the fetus does not consume meals directly, but receives nourishment from the mother via the placenta. The fetal liver releases some blood stem cells that migrate to the fetal thymus, so initially the lymphocytes, called T-cells, are created from fetal liver stem cells. Once the fetus is delivered, the formation of blood stem cells in infants shifts to the red

Chloroquine and Body Tissues

bone marrow. After birth, the umbilical vein and ductus venosus are completely obliterated in two to five days; the former becomes the ligamentum teres and the latter becomes the ligamentum venosum. In the disease state of cirrhosis and portal hypertension, the umbilical vein can open up again.

As food

Liver (food)

Cultural allusions

In Greek mythology, Prometheus was punished by the gods for revealing fire to humans, by being chained to a rock where a vulture (or an eagle) would peck out his liver, which would regenerate overnight. (The liver is the only human internal organ that actually can regenerate itself to a significant extent.) Many ancient peoples of the Near East and Mediterranean areas practiced a type of divination called haruspicy, where they tried to obtain information by examining the livers of sheep and other animals.

In Plato, and in later physiology, the liver was thought to be the seat of the darkest emotions (specifically wrath, jealousy and greed) which drive men to action. The Talmud (tractate *Berakhot 61b*) refers to the liver as the seat of anger, with the gallbladder counteracting this.

The Persian, Urdu, and Hindi languages (جگر or   or *jigar*) refer to the liver in figurative speech to indicate courage and strong feelings, or "their

Chloroquine and Body Tissues

best"; e.g., "This Mecca has thrown to you the pieces of its liver!".[22] The term *jan e jigar*, literally "the strength (power) of my liver", is a term of endearment in Urdu. In Persian slang, *jigar* is used as an adjective for any object which is desirable, especially women. In the Zulu language, the word for liver (isibindi) is the same as the word for courage.

The legend of Liver-Eating Johnson says that he would cut out and eat the liver of each man killed after dinner.

In the motion picture *The Message*, Hind bint Utbah is implied or portrayed eating the liver of Hamza ibn ʻAbd al-Muttalib during the Battle of Uhud. Although there are narrations that suggest that Hind did "taste", rather than eat, the liver of Hamza, the authenticity of these narrations have to be questioned.

GROSS ANATOMY OF SPLEEN

Spleen

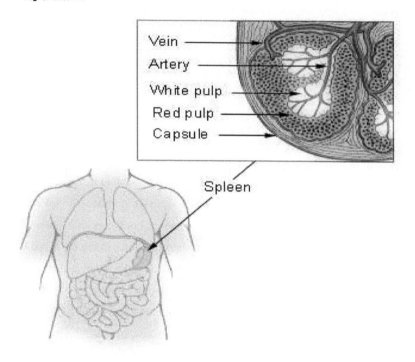

SPLEEN

Chloroquine and Body Tissues

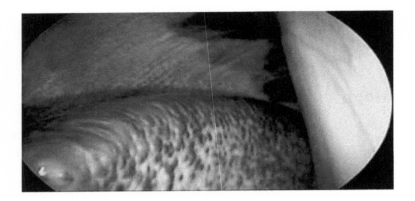

Laparoscopic view of a horse's spleen (the purple and grey mottled organ)

The **spleen** (from Greek σπλήν—*spl̄n*) is an organ found in virtually all vertebrate animals. Similar in structure to a large lymph node, the spleen acts primarily as a blood filter. As such, it is a non-vital organ, with a healthy life possible after removal. The spleen plays important roles in regard to red blood cells (also referred to as erythrocytes) and the immune system. In humans, it is located in the left upper quadrant of the abdomen. It removes old red blood cells and holds a reserve of blood in case of hemorrhagic shock while also recycling iron. As a part of the mononuclear phagocyte system, it metabolizes hemoglobin removed from senescent erythrocytes. The globin portion of hemoglobin is degraded to its constitutive amino acids, and the heme portion is metabolized to bilirubin, which is subsequently shuttled to the liver for removal. It synthesizes antibodies in its white pulp and removes antibody-

Chloroquine and Body Tissues

coated bacteria along with antibody-coated blood cells by way of blood and lymph node circulation. The spleen is brownish. A study published in 2009 using mice showed it has been found to contain in its reserve half of the body's monocytes within the red pulp. These monocytes, upon moving to injured tissue (such as the heart), turn into dendritic cells and macrophages while promoting tissue healing. It is one of the centers of activity of the reticuloendothelial system and can be considered analogous to a large lymph node, as its absence leads to a predisposition toward certain infections.

Anatomy

The spleen, in healthy adult humans, is approximately 11 centimetres (4.3 in) in length. It usually weighs between 150 grams (5.3 oz) and 200 grams (7.1 oz). An easy way to remember the anatomy of the spleen is the $1\times3\times5\times7\times9\times11$ rule. The spleen is 1" by 3" by 5", weighs approximately 7 oz, and lies between the 9th and 11th ribs on the left hand side.

Like the thymus, the spleen possesses only efferent lymphatic vessels. The spleen is part of the lymphatic system. Both the short gastric arteries and the splenic artery supply it with blood.

The germinal centers are supplied by arterioles called *penicilliary radicles.*

The spleen is unique in respect to its development within the gut. While most of the gut viscera are endodermally derived (with the exception of the neural-crest derived suprarenal gland), the spleen is derived from mesenchymal tissue. Specifically, the spleen forms within, and from, the dorsal mesentery. However, it still shares the same blood supply—the celiac trunk—as the foregut organs.

Function

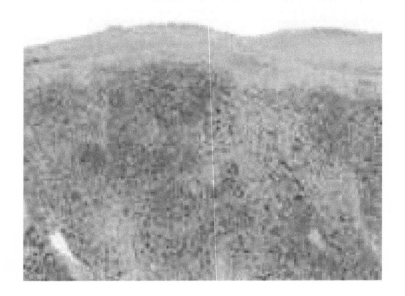

Micrograph of splenic tissue showing the red pulp (red), white pulp (blue) and a thickened inflamed capusule (mostly pink - top of image). H&E stain.

Area	Function	Composition
red pulp	Mechanical filtration of red blood cells. In mice: Reserve of monocytes	• "sinuses" (or "sinusoids"), which are filled with blood • "splenic cords" of reticular fibers • "marginal zone" bordering on white pulp
white pulp	Active immune response through humoral and cell-mediated pathways.	Composed of nodules, called Malpighian corpuscles. These are composed of: • "lymphoid follicles" (or "follicles"), rich in B-lymphocytes • "periarteriolar lymphoid sheaths" (PALS), rich in T-lymphocytes

Other functions of the spleen are less prominent, especially in the healthy adult:

- Production of opsonins, properdin, and tuftsin.
- Creation of red blood cells. While the bone marrow is the primary site of hematopoiesis in the adult, the spleen has important hematopoietic

functions up until the fifth month of gestation. After birth, erythropoietic functions cease, except in some hematologic disorders. As a major lymphoid organ and a central player in the reticuloendothelial system, the spleen retains the ability to produce lymphocytes and, as such, remains an hematopoietic organ.

- Storage of red blood cells, lymphocytes and other formed elements. In horses, roughly 30% of the red blood cells are stored there. The red blood cells can be released when needed. In humans, up to a cup (236.5 ml) of red blood cells can be held in the spleen and released in cases of hypovolemia. It can store platelets in case of an emergency. Up to a quarter of lymphocytes can be stored in the spleen at any one time.
- In mice, the spleen stores half the body's monocytes so that upon injury they can migrate to the injured tissue and transform into dendritic cells and macrophages and so assist wound healing.

Effects of removal

Surgical removal causes:

- modest increases in circulating white blood cells and platelets,
- diminished responsiveness to some vaccines,
- increased susceptibility to infection by bacteria and protozoa; in particular, there is an increased risk of sepsis from polysaccharide encapsulated bacteria.

Chloroquine and Body Tissues

A 28-year follow-up of 740 veterans of World War II who had their spleens removed on the battlefield found that those who had been splenectomized showed a significant excess of mortality from pneumonia (6 rather than the expected 1.3) and a significant excess of mortality from ischemic heart disease (4.1 rather than the expected 3) but not from other conditions.

Disorders

Splenic disease

Disorders include splenomegaly, where the spleen is enlarged for various reasons, such as cancer, specifically blood-based leukemias, and asplenia, where the spleen is not present or functions abnormally.

Etymology and cultural views

The word **spleen** comes from the Greek σπλήν (*spl n*), and is the idiomatic equivalent of the heart in English, i.e. to be good-spleened (εσπλαγχνος , *eúsplankhnos*) means to be good-hearted or compassionate.

In English the word *spleen* was customary during the period of the 18th century. Authors like Richard Blackmore or George Cheyne employed it to characterise the hypocondriacal and hysterical affections. William Shakespeare, in *Julius Caesar* uses the spleen to describe Cassius' irritable nature.

Must I observe you? must I stand and crouch
Under your testy humour? By the gods
You shall digest the venom of your spleen,
Though it do split you; for, from this day forth,
I'll use you for my mirth, yea, for my laughter,
When you are waspish.

In French, "splénétique" refers to a state of pensive sadness or melancholy. It has been popularized by the poet Charles Baudelaire (1821–1867) but was already used before in particular to the Romantic literature (19th century). The word for the organ is "la rate".

The connection between *spleen* (the organ) and *melancholy* (the temperament) comes from the humoral medicine of the ancient Greeks. One of the humours (body fluid) was the black bile, secreted by the spleen organ and associated with melancholy. In contrast, the Talmud (tractate Berachoth 61b) refers to the spleen as the organ of laughter while possibly suggesting a link with the humoral view of the organ. In the eighteenth- and nineteenth-century England, women in bad humour were said to be afflicted by the spleen, or the vapours of the spleen. In modern English, "to vent one's spleen" means to vent one's anger, e.g. by shouting, and can be applied to both males and females. Similarly, the English term "splenetic" is used to describe a person in a foul mood.

Variation among vertebrates

In cartilaginous and ray-finned fish it consists primarily of red pulp and is normally a somewhat elongated organ as it actually lies inside the serosal lining of the intestine. In many amphibians, especially frogs, it takes on the more rounded form and there is often a greater quantity of white pulp.

In reptiles, birds, and mammals, white pulp is always relatively plentiful, and in the latter two groups, the spleen is typically rounded, although it adjusts its shape somewhat to the arrangement of the surrounding organs. In the great majority of vertebrates, the spleen continues to produce red blood cells throughout life; it is only in mammals that this function is lost in the adult. Many mammals possess tiny spleen-like structures known as **haemal nodes** throughout the body, which, it is presumed, have the same function as the spleen proper. The spleens of aquatic mammals are in some ways dissimilar to those of fully land-dwelling mammals. In general, the spleens of aquatic mammals are bluish in colour. In cetaceans and manatees it tends to be quite small, but in deep diving pinnipeds it can be quite massive, owing to its function of storing red blood cells.

The only vertebrates lacking a spleen are the lampreys and hagfishes. Even in these animals, there is a diffuse layer of haematopoeitic tissue within the gut wall, which has a similar structure to red pulp, and is presumed to be homologous with the spleen of higher vertebrates.

Chloroquine and Body Tissues

CHAPTER II

HISTOLOGY

Introduction to Histology

Histology is the microscopic study of the normal tissues of the body whist histopathology is the microscopic study of tissues affected by disease. The procedures adopted for the preparation of material for such studies are known as histological or histopathological techniques and it iswith these techniques that the medical laboratory technician in the pathology department is primarily concerned. The various ways of preparing and examining smears , preserving and processing tissues , cutting and staining sections and the ability to recognize whether or not the procedures have been performed correctly constitute the skills of the medical laboratory scientist in this subject. For the work to be executed competently a knowledge of the structure of cells and the organs and

tissues formed by them is essential . The basic substance of all living things is *protoplasm*, which iscontained within small units , called *cells*, many millions of which go tomake up the human body .Protoplasm is the general name given to the main constituents of a call (of a colloidal nature)together with water, protein, carbohydrates , lipids and inorganic salts. If the cell is studied by histological methods and light microscopy it is seen to contain structures, Electron microscopy, however, shows complete tubular structures in the cytoplasm, and detail in the nucleus not seen by ordinary microscopy.

Chloroquine and Body Tissues

60

The Cell

A cell may be conveniently described as a mass of protoplasm enclosed within a membrane (cell or plasma membrane) containing a subdivision, the nucleus, which is bounded by the nuclear membrane. The portion of cell lying between the plasma and nuclear membranes is known as the cytoplasm. Within the cytoplasm a variety of fine structures called organelles may be identified. These are specialized structures with individual functions and consist of the living material ofthe cell.

Reticular fibers

Structurally similar to collagen fibers to which they are often connected, these fibers differ from collagen in certain methods of demonstration. The delicate networks formed by reticulum fibers offer support for cells, capillaries, and nerve fibers, and are also found at the junctions between connective and other types of tissue.

EXAMINATION OF TUISSUES

Numerous techniques can be used to prepare tissue for microscopical examination, the method selected being governed by a number of factors. These include the structures or inclusions to be studied, the amount and nature of tissue to be examined, whether the specimen is fresh or preserved and the urgency of the investigation.

Fresh specimens

Fresh specimens may be examined as teased and squash preparations, smears, touch preparations or frozen sections.

TEASED PREPARATIONS

These are prepared by carefully dissecting, with mounted needles, the tissue to be examined. The dissection is carried out while the specimen is immersed in an isotonic solution, such as normal saline or Ringer s solution in a petri dish or watch glass. Selected pieces of the tissue are transferred carefully to a microscope slide and mounted as a wet preparation beneath a coverglass, care being taken to avoid the formation of air bubbles. The preparation is then examined by bright filed microscopy, the illumination being reduced either by closing the iris diaphragm or lowering the sub-stage condenser. Many details can be studied in slides prepared by this method, which has the advantage of permitting the cells to be examined in the living state; the preparations,however, are not permanent . The use of the phase contrast microscope greatly increases the structural detail of the cells examined, allowing movement and mitotic division to be observed. The application of certain stains such as methylene blue can be also of great value.

SQUASH PREPARATIONS

The cellular contents of small pieces of tissue not exceeding 1 mm in diameter can be examined by placing the tissue in the center of a microscopic slide and forcibly applying a coverglass. Staining can be carried out if necessary by making use of capillary attraction; a drop of a vital stain placed at the junction of the coverglass and slide is drawn into contact with the tissue which absorbs it.

SMEARS

The microscopic examination of cellular material spread lightly over a slide in the form of a smear is a technique which has wide application in histopathology. The method of preparing the smear differs according to the nature of the material to be examined, but as a general rule smears are made either by spreading the selected portion of the specimen over the surface of the slide with a platinum loop or, alternatively, by making an apposition smear with the aid of a second slide. Smears may be examined either as fresh preparations in a similar manner to that described for teased preparations, or by using a supravital staining technique in conjunction with a warm stage. Both of these techniques suffer from the same disadvantage, namely, that the preparations are permanent. Permanent stained preparations can be made from fresh smears by fixing them while still wet, staining to demonstrate specific structures and inclusions and mounting the cleared specimen beneath a coverglass with a suitable mounting medium.

IMPRESSION SMEARS

These are prepared by bringing into contact the surface of a clean glass slide with that of a freshly cut piece of tissue microscopically by phases contrast or after applying vital stains. Alternatively, the impression smear , which is also

Chloroquine and Body Tissues

known as a touch preparation , can be fixed and stained according to the methods described.

FROZEN SECTIONS

Section of 10-15 um in thickness can be cut from fresh tissue frozen on a microtome with the aid of carbon dioxide or electro-thermal coupling units. The sections are transferred from the microtome knife to a dish containing an isotonic solution , from which they may be either attached to slides prior to staining or carried through the staining solutions by means of a glass rod .

MORPHOLOGY

Morphology - Introduction: (1) Most Plants and Animals Are Aggregates of Cells

So far as living beings have a form and structure, they fall within the province of *Anatomy* and *Histology*, the latter being merely a name for that ultimate optical analysis of living structure which can be carried out only by the aid of the microscope.

And, in so far as the form and structure of any living being are not constant during the whole of its existence, but undergo a series of changes from the commencement of that existence to its end, living beings have a *Development*. The history of development is an account of the anatomy of a living being at the successive periods of its existence, and of the manner in which one anatomical stage passes into the next.

Finally, the systematic statement and generalization of the facts of *Morphology*, in such a manner as to arrange living beings in groups according to their degrees of likeness, is *Taxonomy*.

The study of Anatomy and Development has brought to light certain generalizations of wide applicability and great importance.

It has been said that the great majority of living, beings present a very definite structure. Unassisted vision and ordinary dissection suffice to separate the body of any of the higher animals, or plants, into fabrics of different sorts, which always present the same general arrangement in the organism, but are combined in different ways in different organisms. The discrimination of these comparatively few fabrics, or *tissues*, of which organisms are composed, was the first step towards that ultimate analysis of visible structure which has become possible only by the recent perfection of microscopes and of methods of preparation.

Histology, which embodies the results of this analysis, shows that every tissue of a plant is composed of more or less modified structural elements, each of which is termed a *cell*; which cell, in its simplest condition, is merely a spheroidal mass of protoplasm, surrounded by a coat or sac -- the *cell wall* -- which contains cellulose. In the various tissues, these cells may undergo innumerable modifications of form -- the protoplasm may become differentiated into a nucleus with its nucleolus, a primordial utricle, and a cavity filled with a watery fluid, and the cell-wall may be variously altered in composition or in structure, or may coalesce with others. But, however extensive these changes may be, the fact that the tissues are made up of morphologically distinct units -- the cells -- remains patent. And, it any doubt could exist on the subject, it would be removed by the study of development, which proves that every plant commences its existence as a simple cell, identical in its cells of which the whole body is composed.

But it is not necessary to the morphological unit of the plant that it should be always provided with a cell-wall. Certain plants, such as *Protococcus,* spend longer or shorter periods of their existence in the condition of a mere spheroid of protoplasm, devoid of any cellulose wall, while, at other times, the protoplasmic body becomes enclosed within a cell-wall, fabricated by its superficial layer.

Therefore, just as the nucleus, the primordial utricle, and the central fluid are no essential constituents of the morphological units of the plant, but represent results of its metamorphosis, so the cell-wall is equally unessential; and either the term "cell" must acquire a merely technical significance as the equivalent of morphological unit, or some new term must be invented to describe the latter. On the whole, it is probably least inconvenient to modify the sense of the word "cell".

The histological analysis of animal tissue has led to results and to difficulties of terminology of precisely the same character. In the higher animals, however, the modifications which the cells undergo are so extensive, that the fact that the tissues are, as in plants, resolvable into an aggregation of morphological units, could never have been established without the aid of the study of development, which proves that the animal, no less than the plant, commences its existence as a simple cell, fundamentally identical with the less modified cells which are found in the tissues of the adult.

Though the nucleus is very constant among animal cells, it is not universally present, and among the lowest forms of animal life, the protoplasmic mass which represents the morphological unit may be, as in the lowest plants, devoid of a nucleus. In the animal, the cell-wall, never has the character of a shut sac containing cellulose; and it is not a little difficult, in may cases, to say how much of the so called "cell-wall" of the animal cell answers to the "primordial utricle" and how much to the proper "cellulose cell-wall" of the vegetable cell. But it is certain that in the animal, as in the plant, neither cell-wall nor nucleus are essential constituents of the cell, in as much as bodies which are unquestionably the equivalents of cells -- true morphological units -- are mere masses of protoplasm, devoid alike of cell-wall and nucleus.

For the whole living world, then, it results: -- that the morphological unit -- the primary and fundamental form of life -- is merely an individual mass of protoplasm, in which no further may present but little advance on this

Chloroquine and Body Tissues

structure; and that all the higher forms of life are aggregates of such morphological units or cells, variously modified.

Moreover, all that is at present known tends to the conclusion, that, in the complex aggregates of such units of which all the higher animals and plants consist, no cell has arisen otherwise that by becoming separated from the protoplasm of a pre-existing cell; whence the aphorism "*Omnis cellula e cellula.*"

It may further be added, as a general truth applicable to nucleated cells, that the nucleus rarely undergoes any considerable modification, the structures characteristic of the tissues being formed at the expense of the more superficial protoplasm of the cells; and that, when nucleated cells divide the division of the nucleus, as a rule, precedes that of the whole cell.

STEREOLOGY

Stereology (from Greek stereos = solid) was originally defined as "the spatial interpretation of sections". It is an interdisciplinary field that is largely concerned with the three-dimensional interpretation of planar sections of materials or tissues. It provides practical techniques for extracting quantitative information about a three-dimensional material from measurements made on two-dimensional planar sections of the material (see examples below). Stereology is a method that utilizes random, systematic sampling to provide unbiased and quantitative data. It is an important and efficient tool in many applications of microscopy (such as petrography, materials science, and biosciences including histology, bone and neuroanatomy). Stereology is a developing science with many important innovations being developed mainly in Europe. New innovations such as the proportionator continue to make important improvements in the efficiency of stereological procedures.

In addition to two-dimensional plane sections, stereology also applies to three-dimensional slabs (e.g. 3D microscope images), one-dimensional probes (e.g. needle biopsy), projected images, and other kinds of 'sampling'. It is especially useful when the sample has a lower spatial dimension than the original material. Hence, stereology is often defined as the science of estimating higher dimensional information from lower dimensional samples.

Stereology is based on fundamental principles of geometry (e.g. Cavalieri's principle) and statistics (mainly survey sampling inference). It is a completely different approach from computed tomography.

Classical examples

Classical applications of stereology include:

- calculating the volume fraction of quartz in a rock by measuring the area fraction of quartz on a typical polished plane section of rock ("Delesse principle");

- calculating the surface area of pores per unit volume in a ceramic, by measuring the length of profiles of pore boundary per unit area on a typical plane section of the ceramic (multiplied by $4 / \pi$);
- calculating the total length of capillaries per unit volume of a biological tissue, by counting the number of profiles of capillaries per unit area on a typical histological section of the tissue (multiplied by 2).

The popular science fact that the human lungs have a surface area (of gas exchange surface) equivalent to a tennis court (75 square meters), was obtained by stereological methods. Similarly for statements about the total length of nerve fibres, capillaries etc. in the human body.

Errors in spatial interpretation

The word Stereology was coined in 1961 and defined as `the spatial interpretation of sections'. This reflects the founders' idea that stereology also offers insights and rules for the qualitative interpretation of sections.

Stereologists have helped to detect many fundamental scientific errors arising from the misinterpretation of plane sections. Such errors are surprisingly common. For example:

- plane sections of quenched steel contain thin linear streaks of Martensite. For many years this was interpreted as demonstrating that the Martensite inclusions are "needle-like". But if every plane section

STEREOLOGY TIMELINE

1733 G. Buffon discovers connections between geometry and probability, that ultimately lay the foundations for stereology.

1843 Mining geologist A.E. Delesse invents the first practical technique (Delesse's principle) for determining volume fraction in 3D from area fraction on sections

1885 mathematician M.W. Crofton publishes theory of `geometrical probability' including stereological methods.

1895 first known description of a correct method for counting cells in microscopy.

1898 geologist A. Rosiwal explains how to determine volume fraction from length fraction on linear transects

1916 S.J. Shand builds the first integrating linear accumulator to automate stereological work

1919 committee of ASTM (American Society for Testing and Materials) established to standardise measurement of grain size.

1923 statistician S.D. Wicksell formulates the general problem of particle size - inferring the distribution of sizes of 3-D particles from the observed distribution of sizes of their 2-D profiles - and solves it for spherical particles.

1929 mathematician H. Steinhaus develops stereological principles for measuring length of curves in 2D.

1930-33 geologists A.A. Glagolev and E. Thomson independently propose techniques for determining volume fraction from the ratio of counts of test points.

1940's cancer researcher H. Chalkley publishes methods for determining surface area from plane sections.

1944 mathematician P.A.P. Moran describes a method for measuring the surface area of a convex object from the area of projected images.

1946 anatomist Abercrombie shows that many current methods for counting cells are erroneous, and proposes a correct method

1946–58 materials scientist S.A. Saltykov publishes methods for determining surface area and length from plane sections.

1948 biologist H. Elias uncovers a one-hundred-year-old misunderstanding of the structure of mammalian liver.

1952 Tomkeieff and Campbell calculate the internal surface area of a human lung.

1961 word 'stereology' coined. Foundation of the International Society of Stereology

1961 materials scientists Rhines and De Hoff develop a method for estimating the number of objects e.g. grains, particles, cells of convex shape.

1966 Weibel and Elias calculate the efficiency of stereological sampling techniques.

1972 E. Underwood describes stereological techniques for projected images.

1975-80 statisticians R.E. Miles and P.J. Davy show that stereology can be formulated as a survey sampling technique, and develop design-based methods.

1983 R.E Miles and (independently) E.B. Jensen and H.J.G. Gundersen develop point-sampled intercept methods for inferring the mean volume of arbitrarily-shaped particles from plane sections

1984 D.C Sterio describes the `disector' counting method

1985 stereologist H. Haug criticises the dogma that the normal human brain progressively loses neurons with age. He shows that the existing evidence is invalid.

1985 statistician A. Baddeley introduces the method of vertical sections.

1986 Gundersen proposes the `fractionator' sampling technique

1988-92 Gundersen and Jensen propose the `nucleator' and `rotator' techniques for estimating particle volume.

Chloroquine and Body Tissues

1998 Kubinova introduces the first virtual probe that estimates surface area in preferential slices.

1999 Larsen and Gundersen introduce global spatial sampling for estimation of total length in preferential slices.

2002-05 Mouton and Gokhale introduce "space balls" and "virtual cycloid" for estimation of total length and total surface area, respectively, in preferential slices.

2008 Gundersen, Gardi, Nyengaard introduce the proportionator the most efficient stereological method known. (Gundersen HJ & Jensen EB 2007).

CHAPTER III

EFFECTS OF CHLOROQUINE ON THE KIDNEY,LIVER AND SPLEEN

Abstract

Significant binding of chloroquine occurs in the liver, kidney and spleen
(Taylor and Francis 1987).Hence this study was designed to determine the
effects of administration of chloroquine on the morphology and stereology of
the liver, kidney and spleen. Ten rats were exposed to chloroquine once a day
for three days. The treated rats received the 0.125ml/100g body weight of
chloroquine phosphate injection intraperitineally.Control rats received the
same amount of normal saline intraperitoneally .the histology of the
chloroquine treated kidney, liver and spleen was also compared with controls.
It was observed that chloroquine caused malformation in these tissues.
Histologically, the micrographs of control and treated rats, liver, kidney and
spleen was compared. Investigations confirmed defects in microscopic
structures e.g. for the kidney there were few renal corpuscles in the treated rats
compared with controls. For the liver there were few blood vessels in the
treated rats compared with controls. For the spleen there were few white pulps
in the treated rats compared with controls with controls. Stereologically, the
parameters measured for kidney, liver and spleen was also compared with
controls. The estimated absolute volume V =Vv (structure) x v (ref) of the
blood vessels, renal corpuscles and white pulps of the fractions were
determined and compared. For the liver chloroquine caused a reduction in the

absolute volume of the blood vessels when compared with controls. For the kidney, chloroquine caused a reduction in the absolute volume of the white pulps when compared with control rats

Keywords: chloroquine, liver, kidney, spleen, sprague-dawley rats, stereology, morphology

MATERIALS AND METHODS

Twenty female Sprague- Dawley rats will be collected from the animal house of the college of medicine university of Lagos Akoka, Lagos State.

They will be between 100-150g and will be fed with the normal rat feed from Pfizer PLC Ikeja Lagos. Weight of animals will be taken twice daily throughout the duration of the experiment. Ten female rats will be used as controls. The remaining ten female rats will be labelled by ear puncture as treated rats and kept in cages. Administration of drug was 0.125ml of chloroquine /100g body weight for 3 days intrapertoneally. Chloroquine phosphate injection was obtained from the community pharmacy of the Lagos university teaching hospital (40mg/ml chloroquine phosphate injection).The control received the same quantity of normal saline.

ANIMAL SACRIFICE

At the expiration of the treatment the animals will be sacrificed by diethyl ether decapitation and the liver,kidney, and spleen will be removed for morphological and histological assessment.

HISTOLOGICAL ANALYSIS

The twenty male rats will be sacrificed as discussed earlier after treatment with the chloroquine phosphate injection .The liver, kidney and spleen were removed and fixed in Bouin's fluid. Each specimen of equal length was cut transversely and longitudinally into serial cross sections of 3μm normal thickness with Reichert Jung Supercut Mictrotome for control and treated rats. The tissues were sectioned using tissues preparation tissues method with heamatoxylin and eosin stains and examined the light binocular microscope at a magnification of 100 and 400 respectively.

STEREOLOGICAL ANALYSIS

The vertical sections of the histochemical preparation of stratum length of 0.5cm from 10 control and 10 treated rats liver, kidney, and spleen were made at a final print magnification of 100 and 400 respectively.

5 slides will be obtained from the control and 5 slides from the treated rats.

For each of the fractions, the N/A number of blood vessels, renal corpuscles, per unit area of the fractions were estimated by point counting method using the forbidden rule Hans Gundersen,1977) which states that any structure that touches the forbidden line must not be counted. The reference volume V(ref) of blood vessels, renal corpuscles and white pulps were estimated by point counting (Wiebel, 1979, Gundersen et al, 1988).

Chloroquine and Body Tissues

At Magnification (M) = 100 final magnification using a Square Grid of test point diameter (d) =1.2cm apart. The test system used in the light microscopic analysis within a square frame measuring 20cm x 20cm onto which microscopic image was projected using a wild leitz microscope equipped with a mirror at a magnification of 25 on a white screen.

Estimated V(ref) = (stratum length) x $\underline{d}^2$ x mean N/A (structure).
$$M^2$$

d= diameter of test grid

M=magnification of projection

The relevant volume density of blood vessels, renal corpuscles, and white pulps of the fractions Vv (structure) were estimated on the same section at a final magnification of 100. Each field was projected onto a test system consisting of three sets of points with numerical densities in the ratio 1:4:16. The corresponding distance between the test points of each set were 4.8, 2.4 and 1.2cm respectively.

The criteria for test point design and allocation were based on efficiency considerations; thus approximately the same number of test points (which does not need to exceed 200) should be in each structure within each organ (Gundersen and Jensen, 1987; Gundersen et al ., 1988; Cruz Orive and Wiebel; 1990). The required volume density of the fractions were estimated as follows:

Estimated Vv(structure) = Nv_R x N/A(structure)

Vv = volume density Nv_R = numerical density ratio

Finally, the absolute volume of blood vessels, renal corpuscles and white pulps within each organ was estimated using this equation.

V(structure) =Vv (structure) x V (ref)

V(structure) = absolute volumes of structure

Vv(ref)   = Reference volume of structure

STATISTICS

Statistical analysis was carried out using t- Distribution (t- test).

RESULTS

TABLE 1: ESTIMATED ABSOLUTE VOLUMES (CM^3) OF BLOOD VESSELS RENAL CORPUSCLE AND WHITE PULPS OF CHLOROQUINE TREATED AND CONTROL RATS

TISSUE	CONTROL RATS n=10	CHOLOROQUINE TREATED RATS n=10
Liver (blood vessels)	$4.76 \times 10^{-3} \pm 0.19^a$	$1.93 \times 10\text{-}3 \pm 0.95^b$
Kidney (renal corpuscles)	$4.20 \times 10^{-3} \pm 0.02^a$	$4.15 \times 10\text{-}3 \pm 0.18^b$
Spleen (white pulps)	$5.65 \times 10^{-3} \pm 0.48^a$	$4.0 \times 10\text{-}3 \pm 0.10^b$

a=Mean±S.E.M   b=$p<0.05$

TABLE2: MEAN NUMBER OF BLOOD VESSELS PER UNIT AREA (N/A)

GROUP n=20	MEAN (N/A)
CONTROL (CO)	3.0
TREATED(CQ)	1.0

CO =CONTROL CQ =CHLOROQUINE TREATED RATS

Chloroquine and Body Tissues

TABLE3: MEAN NUMBER OF RENAL CORPUSCLES PER UNIT AREA (N/A)

GROUP n=20	MEAN (N/A)
CONTROL(CO)	2.0
TREATED(CQ)	1.8

CO =CONTROL CQ =CHLOROQUINE TREATED RATS

TABLE 4: MEAN NUMBER OF WHITE PULPS PER UNIT AREA (N/A)

GROUP n=20	MEAN N/A
CONTROL (CO)	1.5
TREATED (CQ)	2.0

CO =CONTROL   CQ =CHLOROQUINE TREATED RATS

Chloroquine and Body Tissues

DISCUSSION

HISTOMORPHOMETRIC EFFECTS

Chloroquine caused defects in the microscopic structure of the liver kidney and spleen of the Sprague-Dawley rats. Renal corpuscles were few and deformed with noticeable patches in the kidney when compared with controls. Blood vessels in the treated rats compared with controls were few in the liver when compared with controls. They were few white pulps in the treated rats spleen compared with controls. Stereologically, the individual estimated absolute volume of fractions were determined and compared. For the liver there was a reduction in the absolute volume of the blood vessels when compared with controls. For the kidney, Chloroquine caused a reduction in the absolute volume of the renal corpuscles when compared with controls. Lastly for the spleen chloroquine caused a reduction in the absolute volume of the white pulps when compared with controls.

HISTOLOGY

This study focused on the microscopic structures of the liver, kidney and spleen of animals treated with chloroquine once a day for three days. The investigation confirmed defects in microscopic structures. For the kidney, there were few renal corpuscles with noticeable patches in the treated rats compared with controls .for the liver there were few blood vessels in the treated rats compared with controls. For the spleen there were few white pulps in the treated rats compared with controls (Patricia & Nathan, 1981).

STEREOLOGY

This study focused on the morphometric investigations. Absolute volumes of the liver, kidney and spleen special components were stereologically estimated after treatment with chloroquine. The investigation confirmed that chloroquine has deleterious effects on the quantitative analysis of these important tissues of the body (Ausburger & Arnold 1991).There was a reduction in the absolute volume of the blood vessels present in the liver after treatment with chloroquine compared with controls. There was a reduction in the absolute volume of the renal corpuscles after chloroquine treatment compared with controls. There was a reduction in the absolute volume of white pulps after chloroquine treatment compared with controls. (Cruz-Orive et al 1993).

CONCLUSION AND SUMMARY

In summary the present study has demonstrated that chloroquine though an antimalaria drug when taken in the rightful dosage have deleterious effects on some vital organs in the body. Chloroquine has deleterious effects on the microscopic structures of the liver, kidney and spleen and on the morphometric /quantitative analysis of the liver, kidney and spleen vital components. However, further research are necessary on these findings.

BIBLIOGRAPHY

1. Adelusi S.A et al (1982) protein binding of chloroquine in the presence of Aspirin J Clin   Pharmacol 13 (3):451-452

2. Asaoka K.,Ito H& Tisell (1980): Morphology of rats prostate lobes and seminal vesicles after long –term estrogen treatment Acta Pathol Microbial Immunol Scand (A) 90:441-448

3. Augsburger.H,U Farber (1991): Morphological basis of urinary continence Anat Hist Embryol 20:265

4. Author et al (1976) Childhood chloroquine poisoning – Wisconsin and Washington et al. Journal of the American Association 260:1361

5. Berg T, DeLanghe S, Al Alam D, Utley S, Estrada J, Wang KS (2010). "β-catenin regulates mesenchymal progenitor cell differentiation during hepatogenesis". *J Surg Res* **164** (2): 276–85

6. Bramstedt K (2006). "Living liver donor mortality: where do we stand?". *Am. J. Gastrointestinal* **101** (4): 755–9.Brender, MD, Erin; Allison Burke, MA, illustrator, Richard M. Glass, MD, editor (2005-11-23). "Spleen Patient Page" (PDF). *Journal of the American Medical Association* (American Medical Association) **294** (20): 2660.

8. Bunnag, D., Harinasuta, T . (1987): Quinine and quinidine in malaria in Thailand Acta Leidansia 55:163-166

9. Charles M; Wool .F (1968) Principles of biometry 1:1-350

10.Charoasia B.D (1980) Human anatomy 3: 200-250

Chloroquine and Body Tissues

11. Chen-Pan C, Pan IJ, Yamamoto Y, Sakogawa T, Yamada J, Hayashi Y. Prompt recovery of damaged adrenal medullae induced by salinomycin.Toxicol Pathol. 1999 Sep-Oct;27(5):563-72.

12. Cope, G.H (1979) stereological analysis of the duct system of the rabbit parotid gland J.Anat 126:591-604

13. Cruz-Orive, L.M. E.R Weibel (1990): Recent stereological methods for cell biology : A brief survey Am J Physio 258: L 148-L156

14. Dai J, Han Y, Xu B, Li Y, Liu J, Zhao Y, Zhang F. Ultrastructural changes of nucleoli in common wheat induced by actinomycin D.Biotech Histochem. 2005 Sep-Dec;80(5-6):223-5.

15. Elias, H., D.M Hyde, R. L Scheaffer (1983): A guide to practical stereology Am J Anat 159 :500-580

16. Elias, H., D.M, Hyde (1980): Elementary stereology am J Anat 159 : 411-446

17. Framcos T.F et al (1973) Life depend on the liver 1: 50-57

18. Gannon M.C et al (1997) Diabetologic 40 (70) 758-763

19. Gundersen, H.I.G.,E.B.Jesen (1987): The efficiency of systematic sampling in stereology and its prediction J.Microse 147:229-263

20. Gundersen, H.J.G., T.F.Bentsen. L.Korbo, N. Marcussen, A. Moller.K. Nielsen. J.R. Nyengaard, B. Pakkenberg. F.B Sorensen. A. Veterby, M.J West (1988): Some new, simple and efficient stereological methods and their use pathological research and diagnosis APMIS 96:379-394

21. Hollingdaje, M.R. (1985): Malaria and the liver. Hepatology 5:327 -335

Chloroquine and Body Tissues

22. Iwadare T, Harada E, Yoshino S, Arai T: A solution for removal of resin from epoxy sections. *Stain Technol* 1990, 65:205-209.

23. Jia, T.; Pamer, E. G. (2009). "Dispensable but Not Irrelevant". *Science* **325** (5940): 549–550.

24. Koranda F.C (1981) : Antimalaria Journal Of The American Academy Of Dermatology 4 (6) :650-655

25. Li C, Yang S, Chen L, Lu W, Qiu X, Gundersen HJ, Tang Y. Stereological methods for estimating the myelin sheaths of the myelinated fibers in white matter.Anat Rec (Hoboken). 2009 Oct;292(10):1648-55.

26. Lori Sheporaitis; Patrick C. Freeney. *Hepatic and Portal Surface Veins:A New Anatomic Variant Revealed During Abdominal CT.* American Journal of Roengenology 1998;171:1559-1564.

27. Loty et al (1982) Comparison of the effects of chronic chloroquine treatment and derivation on noradrenergic mechanisms J Med Bio L60 (1) :23 -25

28. Machiney J.L.S et al (1981) Malaria breakthroughs and resistance to chloroquine in Africa Afr Med J 60 (20) 786-788

29. Mitsui Y, Schmelzer JD, Zollman PJ, Mitsui M, Tritschler HJ, Low PA: Alpha-lipoic acid provides neuroprotection from ischemia-reperfusion injury after peripheral nerve. *J Neurol Sci* 1999, 163:11-16.

30. Patricia .A Dennis and Nathan N. Aronson J.R (1981) Effects of low temperature and chloroquine on I^{125} , insulin degradation by the

perfused rat liver . Archives of Biochemistry and Biophysics 212:170-176

31. Spielmann, Audrey L.; David M. DeLong, Mark A. Kliewer (1 January 2005). "Sonographic Evaluation of Spleen Size in Tall Healthy Athletes". *American Journal of Roentgenology* (American Roentgen Ray Society) **2005** (184): 45–49.

32. Suzuki K, Tanaka M, Watanabe N, Saito S, Nonaka H, Miyajima A (July 2008). "p75 Neurotrophin receptor is a marker for precursors of stellate cells and portal fibroblasts in mouse fetal liver". *Gastroenterology* **135** (1): 270–281.

33. Swirski, F. K.; Nahrendorf, M.; Etzrodt, M.; Wildgruber, M.; Cortez-Retamozo, V.; Panizzi, P.; Figueiredo, J. -L.; Kohler, R. H. et al. (2009). "Identification of Splenic Reservoir Monocytes and Their Deployment to Inflammatory Sites". Science **325** (5940): 612–616.

34. Turgut M, Uyanıkgil Y, Baka M, Tunc AT, Yavasoglu A, Yurtseven ME, Kaplan S: Pinealectomy exaggerates and melatonin treatment suppresses neuroma formation of transected sciatic nerve in rats: gross morphological, histological and stereological analysis. Science 325 (5940): 612–616.

35. Turgut M, Uysal A, Pehlivan M, Oktem G, Yurtseven ME: Assessment of effects of pinealectomy and exogenous melatonin administration on rat sciatic nerve suture repair: an electrophysiological, electron microscopic, and immunohistochemical study. Anat Rec (Hoboken). 2009 Oct;292(10):1648-55.

36. Turgut M, Yenisey C, Uysal A, Bozkurt M, Yurtseven ME: The effects of pineal gland transplantation on the production of spinal deformity and serum melatonin level following pinealectomy in the chicken.

37. Vellguth, Swantje; Brita von Gaudecker, Hans-Konrad Müller-Hermelink. "The development of the human spleen". Cell and Tissue Research (Springer Berlin / Heidelberg) **242** (3): 579–592.

38. Xu Q-G, Zochodne DW: Ischemia and failed regeneration in chronic experimental neuromas. Brain Res 2002, 946:24-30.

39. Yu W, Kauppila T, Hultenby K, Persson JKE, Xu XJ, Wiesenfeld-Hallin Z: Photochemically-induced ischemic injury of the rat sciatic nerve: a light- and electron microscopic study Biological Psychiatry, 35, 501 -516.

40. Zatsepina OV, Voronkova LN, Sakharov VN, Chentsov YS. Ultrastructural changes in nucleoli and fibrillar centers under the effect of local ultraviolet microbeam irradiation of interphase culture cells.Exp Cell Res. 1989 Mar;181(1):94-104.

41. Zhang S, Bodenreider O. Law and order: assessing and enforcing compliance with ontological modeling principles in the Foundational Model of Anatomy.Comput Biol Med. 2006 Jul-Aug;36(7-8):674-93.

42. Zhang W, Li C, Yang S, Xu C, Wang W, Nyengaard JR, Tang Y. A stereological method for estimating the total length and size of myelinated fibers in rat cerebral cortex.J Neurosci Methods. 2008 Jul 15;172(1):21-6. Epub 2008 Apr 14.

43. Zipursky, R.B., Marsh, L., Lim, K.O., *et al* (1994) *Volumetric MRI assessment of temporal lobe structures in schizophrenia.* Biological Psychiatry, 35, 501 -*516.*

44. Zyss R, Gajkowska B. Changes in the function and fine structure of the chromaffin cells of rat adrenal medulla after burn.Pol Med J. 1972;11(2):405-14.

APPENDICES

SOME IMPOTANT MEDICAL TERMS AND THEIR DEFINITIONS

A

A band: Dark band seen in muscle which is made of the thick filaments

Acetylcholine: One of the neurotransmitters

Acidophilia: Property of tissues with an affinity for acidic dye

Acidophils: Cell type in the adenohypophysis with a propensity for acidic dyes

Acinar cell: Cell lining an acinus, such as cells in a pancreatic acini

Acinus: Sac-like cluster of secretory epithelial cells with a central lumen

Acoustic hair cell: Sensory cell within the organ of corti

Acrosome: Portion of a sperm which contains enzymes

Actin:A contractile protein that is very prevalent in muscle

Adenosine triphosphate:A molecule that stores chemical energy; often abbreviated as ATP

Adipocyte: Fat cell

Adipose cell: Fat cell

Adipose: Fatty

Adventitia: The outer connective tissue covering of an organ, vessel or other structure

Agranulocytes: Agranular leukocyte. Leukocytes without prominent granules; specifically lymphocytes and monocytes

Alpha cell:1. Pancreatic islet cell which secrete glucagon

2. Cell type in the anterior pituitary, also called acidophil

Alveolar cell: Cell of the pulmonary alveoli

Alveolar duct: Passageway which contains alveolar sacs

Alveolar sac: Region at the end of an alveolar duct; airspace

Alveolus:1. Microscopic sac in the lung 2. Spherical sac

Amacrine cells: Interneurons in the retina

Ameloblast: Cell which makes tooth enamel

Ampulla:A saccular swelling

Antrum: Fluid filled space surrounding follicle

Apocrine gland:A type of sweat gland found in the axilla, anogenital region, external auditory meatus and eyelid

APUD: Amine precursor uptake and decarboxylation

Argentaffin cells: Also called enterochromaffin cells; found in glands of the gastrointestinal tract; stain with silver salt

Argyrophilic cell: Small granule cell or dense core granule cell

Arrector pili: Smooth muscle associated with a hair follicle

Arteriole: Part of the arterial tree; a small artery with a diameter less than .5mm

Astrocyte: Star shaped cell seen in the central nervous systm; most abundant glial cell

Auerbach's plexus: Myenteric plexus; located in the muscle of the intestine between the outer longitudinal layer and inner circular layer

Axolemma: Plasma membrane of an axon

Axon: Single process seen in a neuron which conducts impulses away from the

Chloroquine and Body Tissues

cell body

Axon hillock: The cone shaped region at the junction of the axon and cell body

Azurophilic granules: Granules in a neutrophil which contain peroxidase and lysosomal enzymes

Abdominal pain: Pain in the belly. Abdominal pain can be acute or chronic. It may reflect a major problem with one of the organs in the abdomen, such as appendicitis or a perforated intestine, or it may result from a fairly minor problem, such as excess buildup of intestinal gas.

Abdominal: Relating to the abdomen, the belly, that part of the body that contains all of the structures between the chest and the pelvis. The abdomen is separated anatomically from the chest by the diaphragm, the powerful muscle spanning the body cavity below the lungs.

See the entire definition of Abdominal

Abductor: (L. abducere, to move away). A muscle that draws a structure away from the axis of the body or one of its parts, e.g. lateral rectus muscle.

Accessorius (L. accessorius, to move toward). Accessory or supernumerary. Also denoting specific muscles.

Accessory: (L. accessorius, to move toward). Supernumerary, adjuvant.

Acetaminophen: A nonaspirin pain reliever or analgesic. Acetaminophen may be given alone to relieve pain and inflammation or it may be combined with other drugs, as in some migraine medications, which contain acetaminophen, a barbiturate, and caffeine.

Adductor:(L. adducere, to bring forward). A muscle that draws a structure toward the axis of the body or one of its parts, e.g. adductor pollicis.

Alae: (L. ala, wing).Relating to a muscle of the nose, and others.

Allergic reaction: The hypersensitive response of the immune system of an allergic individual to a substance

Ameba: A single-celled, protozoan organism that constantly changes shape. Amebae can infect the bowels, causing diarrhea. They can also infect the liver, causing abscesses to form.

Anconeus:(G. ankon, elbow). Musculus anconeus.

Anemia: A reduction in the number of circulating red blood cells or in the quantity of hemoglobin.

Ani:(L. anus, anal oriface). Pertaining to a muscle that supports the anus.

*Anopheles***:** A genus of mosquito, some species of which can transmit human malaria.

Anorexia: Lack of appetite, lack of desire or interest in food.

Anthropophilic: Describes mosquitoes that prefer to take blood meals from humans.

Antibiotic: A drug that kills or slows the growth of bacteria. Example: penicillin.

Antibody: A specialized serum protein (immunoglobulin or gamma globulin) produced by B lymphocytes in the blood in response to an exposure to foreign proteins ("antigens"). The antibodies specifically bind to the antigens that induced the immune response. Antibodies help defend the body against infectious agents such as bacteria, viruses or parasites.

Anticus: (L. anticus, anterior). Designating a muscle as placed anteriorly, e.g. serratus anterior.

Antigen: Any substance that stimulates the immune system to produce antibodies. Antigens are often foreign substances such as parts of invading bacteria, viruses or parasites.

Antimicrobial agents: The drugs, chemicals, or other substances that kill or slow the growth of microbes. They include antibacterial drugs (which kill bacteria), antiviral agents (which kill viruses), antifungal agents (which kill fungi), and antiparasitic drugs (which kill parasites).

Antimicrobial resistance: Antimicrobial resistance is the result of microbes changing in ways that reduce or eliminate the effectiveness of drugs, chemicals, or other agents to cure or prevent infections.

Aralen: A brand name for chloroquine phosphate.

Arch:(L. arcus, a bow). Any structure resembling a bent bow or an arch.

Artemisinins: A class of drugs used for the treatment (not prevention) of malaria usually as a part of a combination therapy, derived from the sweet wormwood or Qinghao plant (*Artemisia annua*).

Articulationis:(L. articulationes, the forming of new joints of a vine). Pertaining to muscles that insert into a joint capsule.

Arytenoid: (G. arytenoideus, ladel-shaped). Pertaining to muscles attached to this laryngeal cartilage.

Atlanto-(G. Atlas, in Greek mythology a Titan who supported the world on his shoulders). Relating to muscles attached to the second cervicle vertebra, the atlas.

Atloideus: See Atlanto-

Atovaquone: A drug used against malaria. It is found in the combination atovaquone-proguanil which can be used for both prevention and treatment.

Audit trail: A sequence of records, each of which contains evidence or other forms of knowledge pertaining to and resulting from the execution of a process or system function. In the *morphological modelling* process it is the definitions of the *parameters* and *parameter values*, and the recording of the reasoning behind each of the *Cross-consistency assessments*.

Auricularis:(L. auricularis, the external ear). Pertaining to muscles that attach to the external ear. Also referring to the fifth digit of the hand because of its use in cleaning the external auditory meatus.

Autochthonous: Regarding malaria, it refers to local transmissionÂ by mosquitoes.Â This can either be indigenous (a geographic area where malaria occurs regularly) or introduced (in a geographic area where malaria does not occur regularly).

Axillary: (L. axilla, armpit). Pertaining to muscles that are found in the region of the armpit, e.g. axillary arch muscle.

Azygos:(G. a, without + zygon, yoke). Any unpaired muscle.

Abdomen. The third, posterior major division of the body. In ants, this also includes the propodeum, which is fused to the thorax and appears to be a thoracic segment, as well as the petiole and postpetiole (if present) found between the propodeum and the gaster.

Aciculate. Finely striate, as if scratched by a needle.

Acidopore. The orifice of the formic acid projecting system found in the subfamily Formicinae. It is formed from the apex of the Hypopygium and usually appears as a short nozzle, generally fringed with short setae at its apex.

Acuminate. Tapering to a fine point.

Acute. Sharply angulate (less than 90 degrees)

Aedeagus. The penis.

Alate. Winged, both males and queens may have wings.

Alitrunk. The second, middle major division of the body. It consists of the thorax (the true thorax) and the first segment of the true abdomen (the propodeum), which is fused to the rear of the thorax. The alitrunk is sometimes called the mesosoma.

Alveolate. Honeycombed and with alveoli (cup shaped depressions) each of which contain a hair.

Anal cell. The space between the anal veins.

Antenna (plural: antennae). One of the paired, flexible, segmented sensory appendages on the head. The antenna consists of an elongate basal segment, the scape, followed distally by 3-11 smaller segments, which taken together form the funiculus.

Antennal condyles. The narrowed, neck-like portions of the first antennal segment that connect to the head surface.

Antennal fossa. The cavity or depression of the head where the antenna is articulated from.

Antennal scrobe. A groove, impression, or excavation found on the side of the head running above or below the eye that accommodates the antennal scape and sometimes the entire antenna.

Antennomere. Antennal segment.

Anterior tentorial pits. A pair of pits or impressions found anteriorly on the dorsal surface of the head, at or near the posterior clypeal margin. The pits indicate the points of attachment of the anterior arms of the internal skeleton (tentorium) of the head to the head capsule.

Apical. At or near the tip.

Appressed. Referring to a hair running parallel or almost parallel to the body surface.

Arcuate. Curved, bow-like.

Areolate. Being divided into a number of small and irregular spaces or cavities.

Arolium (plural: arolia). Pad-like structure found between the tarsal claws.

B

B lymphocytes: Leukocytes involved in humoral immunity

Band cell: Immature neutrophil in which the nucleus has not yet become multilobulated

Barr body: Inactive, repressed X chromosome seen in the female

Basal body: Structure at the base of cilium or flagellum made of microtubules

Basal cell: Cell in the deepest layer of epithelium

Basal lamina: Thin sheet of protein underlying epithelium

Basement membrane: Thin sheet which cells rests upon

Basket cell:1. Cell in the cerebellar cortex 2. Myoepithelial cell

Basophil:1. Type of granulocyte with prominent basophilic granules
2. Glandular cell in the pituitary

Basophilia:1. An increase number of basophils in the peripheral circulation 2. Tissues property of staining with basic dyes

Beta cell: 1. Pancreatic islet cell which secretes insulin 2. Cell type in the anterior pituitary, also called basophil

Betz cells: Pyramidal cells in the motor area of the brain

Bipolar neuron: Neuron with only two processes: an axon and a dendrite

Bowman's capsule: Portion of the uriniferous tubule; double layered portion surrounding the glomeruli

Bowman's membrane: The basement membrane of the corneal epithelium

Bronchiole: Small branch of the bronchial tree which contains no cartilage in the wall

Bruch's membrane: The inner layer of the choroid; also called lamina vitrea

Brunner's gland: Glands found in the submucosa of the duodenum which have an alkaline secretion

Brush border: Microvilli seen on the epithelial surface in the small intestine which significantly increases the absorptive surface area

Bacteria: (singular: Bacterium) Single-celled organisms that are found throughout nature and can be beneficial or cause disease.

Basilaris:(G., L., basis, base). Pertaining to the base, body, or lower part of a structure, e.g., base of the skull.

B-cell (B-lymphocyte): White blood cells of the immune system that are derived from the bone marrow and spleen. B cells develop into plasma cells, which produce antibodies.

Biceps:(L. bi, two + caput, head). Two heads. Pertaining to muscles with two heads, e.g., biceps brachii.

Biventer:(L. bi, two + venter, belly). Muscle having two bellies.

Blindness: Loss of useful sight. Blindness can be temporary or permanent. Damage to any portion of the eye, the optic nerve, or the area of the brain responsible for vision can lead to blindness. There are numerous (actually, innumerable) causes of blindness. The current politically correct terms for blindness include visually handicapped and visually challenged.

Blurred vision: Lack of sharpness of vision with, as a result, the inability to see fine detail. Blurred vision can occur when a person who wears corrective lens is without them. Blurred vision can also be an important clue to eye disease.

Brachialis:(G. brachion, arm). Muscles relating to the arm.

Brachii:(G. brachion, arm). Muscles of the arm.

Brachio-(G. brachion, arm) Relating to the arm.

Breathing: The process of respiration, during which air is inhaled into the lungs through the mouth or nose due to muscle contraction and then exhaled due to muscle relaxation.

Brevis:(L. brevis, short, brief).A short muscle or head, e.g., short head of biceps brachii.

Buccinator:(L. buccinator, trumpeter). A muscle of the cheek.

Bucco-(L. bucca, cheek) Pertaining to the cheek.

Bulbo-(L. bulbus, a bulbus root). Any globular or fusiform structurs. A muscle covering a bulbar structure.

Basal lamella. A thin strip of cuticle found on the apical margin proximal to any teeth that may be present.

Basitarsus. First segment of the tarsus.

Bidentate. Bearing two teeth.

Buccal cavity. Mouth cavity.

C

C cells:1. Parafollicular cells in the thyroid which secrete calcitonin

2. Chromophobe cells of the anterior pituitary

Canal of Schlemm: Circular canal near the junction of the cornea and sclera which allows the aqueous humor to drain from the anterior chamber

Canaliculi: Little canals which contain the processes of an osteocyte

Canals of Hering: Small bile ducts which connect to bile ducts in the portal canal

Cancellous bone: Spongy bone; trabecular bone

Capillary: Thin walled blood vessel; the exchange of products between the blood and tissue occurs in the capillary

Caveola: Small pockets or indentations of cell membrane seen with

Chloroquine and Body Tissues

pinocytosis

Cell membrane: Plasmalemma; outermost portion of of a cell

Cementum: Substance found covering the roots of teeth

Central vein: Vein within the center of a liver lobule

Centriole: Organelle in cells which is made of microtubles

Chief cells:1. Cells in the stomach which secrete pepsinogen 2. Cell type found in the parathyroid

Chondroblast: Immature cartilage cell which forms cartilage

Chondrocyte: Mature cartilage cell

Choroid: Pigmented layer underneath the neural retina

Chromaffin cells: Catacholamine secreting cells found primarily in the adrenal medulla

Chromatin:DNA and histone protein which is found in the cell nucleus

Chromophobe: Cell type in the anterior pituitary which does not pick up stain readily

Chromosome: Structure visible during cell division; bar like structure of chromatin

Capsularis:(L. capsa, a chest or box). A muscle joined to a capsule as, for example, a joint. Any structure so designated as a capsule.

Carbamate: A chemical product used as an insecticide.

Cardiac: Having to do with the heart.

Carina. Elevated ridge or keel.

Carinate. Having carinae, especially in parallel rows.

Carinula. A small carina.

Chloroquine and Body Tissues

Cephalic. Pertaining to the head.

Clavate, claviform. Thickened, especially near or at the tip.

Clypeus (plural: clypei). The foremost section fob the head, just behind the mandibles and demarcated posteriorly by a transverse suture.

Condyle. A structure that articulates any appendage to the body surface.

Cordate. Heart-shaped.

Corrugated. Wrinkled with alternative and parallel ridges and channels.

Costa. A ridge or keel that is rounded at the top.

Costate. Having costae, especially in parallel rows.

Costula. A small costa.

Costulate. Having costulae, especially in parallel rows.

Coxa (plural: coxae). The basal, or first segment of the leg, that attaches the leg to the body.

Carma: *Computer Aided Resource for Morphological Analysis*: The Software system used for carrying out morphological modelling and creating morphological inference models.

Carnosus:(L. carnis, flesh or muscle). Pertaining to muscular tissue or dermal muscles.

Carpi:(G. karpos, wrist). Muscles relating to the eight carpal bones of the wrist.

Caudatus:(L. cauda, tail) The belly of a muscle. When the bellies are divided, bicaudatus.

Cavernosus:(L. caverna, a grotto or hollow). Pertaining to the cavernous tissue of the reproductive system.

Cerato-(G. keras, horn). Relating to muscle that arises from the greater horn of the hyoid bone.

Cerebral malaria: A severemalaria syndrome in which infected red blood cells obstruct blood circulation in the small blood vessels in the brain and/or release cytokines that disrupt normal brain function.

Chemoprophylaxis: The use of antimalarial drugs to prevent malaria disease.

Chills: feelings of coldness accompanied by shivering. Chills may develop after exposure to a cold environment or may accompany a fever.

Chloroquine: A drug used against malaria for both prevention and treatment. A very safe and inexpensive drug, its value has been compromised by the emergence of chloroquine-resistant malaria parasites.

Chondro-(G. chondros, cartilage). Pertaining to muscles that arise from costal cartilage.

Cilia: Hair like projection found on the apical surface of some epithelium

Clara cell: Cells found in the epithelium of the lung

Collagen: Protein found in connective tissue, skin, tendon, bone, and cartilage

Collecting duct: Part of the kidney which collects urine from the nephrons

Columnar cell: An epithelial cell that is taller than it is wide

Compound gland:A gland with branching ducts

Cone cell: Type of photoreceptor which is specialized for color vision

Cords of Billroth: The tissue between the splenic sinuses; also called the splenic cords

Corona radiata: Cell layer surrounding oocyte

Corpus albicans: White scar seen when the corpus luteum degenerates

Corpus luteum: Structure seen in the ovary at site of ruptured follicle; yellow body

Crypts of Lieberkühn: Glands found in the epithelium of the small intestine

Cuboidal epithelium: Type of epithelium where the cells are as tall as they are wide

Cumulus oophorus: Cells which surround the ovum within the ovarian follicle

Cytokinesis: Division of the cytoplasm

Cytoplasm: The region of a cell between the nucleus and plasma membrane

Cytoskeleton: The framework of a cell

Capitis:(L. caput, head). Pertaining to the head.

Cilii:(L. cilium, eyelid). Pertaining to the eyebrow, e.g., corrigator supercilii.

Cinchonism: Side effects from quinine or quinidine. Includes tinnitus, headache, nausea, diarrhea, altered auditory acuity, and blurred vision. The term derives from cinchona bark, the natural source of quinine.

Clavicularis:(L. clavicula, small key). Pertaining to muscles associated with the clavicle.

Cleido-(G. kleis, clavicle). Related with the clavicle.

Clindamycin: An antibiotic that can be used for the treatment of malaria in combination with a second drug, usually quinineÂ or quinidine.

Clinical cure: Elimination of malaria symptoms, sometimes without eliminating all parasites. See "radical cure" and "suppressive cure/treatment."

Coccygeus.(G. kokkyx, a cuckoo). A muscle associated with the coccyx, e.g., musculus coccygeus.

Coherence: Degree of interconnection and consistency between parts - in this case between the *parameter values* in a morphological field.

Colli:(L. collum, neck). Pertaining to the neck or to the neck of a structure, e.g., longus colli muscle.

Coma: A decreased state of consciousness from which a person cannot be roused.

Coma: A state of deep, unarousable unconsciousness. A coma may occur as a result of head trauma, disease, poisoning, or numerous other causes. Coma states are sometimes graded based on the absence or presence of reflexive responses to stimuli.

Communis:(L. communis, in common). Relating to more than one structure working as one unit, e.g., extensor digitorum communis.

Complex Adaptive System (CAS): In social science, a dynamic (dispersed and decentralized) network of agents (e.g. individuals, organisations, institutions, nations) acting concurrently and reacting to each other.

Compressor:(L. compressus, to press together). A muscle that, when contracted, produces pressure on another structure.

Conditions: (see also "Parameter Values"): The different states or values a parameter can take; the parameter's value range

Condyloideus:(G. kondylos, knuckle). Pertaining to a muscle attached to the outer edge of a joint or a bony knob-like stucture.

Configuration cluster: A Collection of configurations, all of which are consistent with a given (selected) condition (see Diagram 3)

Configuration: At least one parameter value or condition displayed from each of the parameters in a morphological model

Congenital malaria: Malaria in a newborn or infant, transmitted from the mother.

Consistency: Degree of compatibility between statements or conditions; in this case between the *conditions* of different *parameters* in a *morphological field.*

Constrictor:(L. constringere). A muscle that, upon contraction, reduces the size of a canal, a sphincter.

Contextual Environment: Those processes and conditions in the outside world, which can influence our organisation, but which we cannot influence significantly ("External world factors").

Coraco-(G. korakoides, a crow's beak). Denoting a muscle that arises from the coracoid process of the scapula.

Cornu:(L. cornu, horn). Any structure resembling a horn in shape.

Corrugator:(L. con, together + ruga, wrinkel). A muscle that wrinkels the skin.

Costalis:(L. costa, rib). Pertaining to muscles attached to ribs.

Cremaster:(G. kremaster, a suspender). Musculus cremaster, the muscle by which the testicles are suspended.

Crico-(G. kikos, a ring). Denoting muscles that attach to the cricoid cartilage.

Cross Consistency Assessment - CCA: Pertains to the process by which the *parameter values* (or parameter *conditions*) in the *morphological field* are compared with one another, pair-wise, in the manner of a cross-impact matrix

Crural:(L. crus, leg). Pertaining to the leg (from knee to ankle) or to any other muscle designated as a crus.

Cryptic malaria: A case of malaria where epidemiologic investigations fail to identify an apparent mode of acquisition (this term applies mainly to cases found in non-endemic countries).

Cure: 1. To heal, to make well, to restore to good health. Cures are easy to claim and, all too often, difficult to confirm. 2. A time without recurrence of a disease so that the risk of recurrence is small, as in the 5-year cure rate for malignant melanoma.

D

Dealate. Having shed the wings.

Declivity. Downward sloping surface, such as the posterior face of the propodeum.

Decumbent. Referring to a hair standing 10 to 40 degrees from the body surface.

Dentate. Toothed, as in the dentate inner borders of mandible.

Denticulate. With minute teeth or tooth-like structures.

Depressed. Flattened down.

Diastema. A relatively large and obvious gap between two adjacent teeth on the mandible.

Distal. Farthest away from body.

Dorsal. Upper surface, the dorsum.

Dorsoventral. Along a line drawn from the upper to lower surface.

Dorsum. Upper surface.

Decidual cell: Cell type in the endometrial stroma

Delta cell:1. Pancreatic islet cell which secretes somatostatin 2. Gonadotrophic cell

Demilune: Crescent shaped serous cell cap seen in some salivary glands

Dendrite: Processes extending from the neuron cell body which usually branch like a tree

Dense core granule cell: Small granule cell or argyrophilic cell

Dense irregular connective tissue: Type of connective tissue where the collagen fibers are in a haphazard arrangement

Dense regular connective tissue: Connective tissue with collagen fibers in parallel arrangement

Dentin: The substance which makes up most of a tooth

Dermis: The layer of skin underneath the epidermis composed primarily of dense irregular connective tissue

Descemet's membrane: Limiting layer of cornea

Desmosome: Type of cell junction; important juction within epithelial tissue; macula adherens

Distal convoluted tubule:DCT; part of the nephron

DNA: Deoxyribonucleic acid; material which carries the genetic information

Ducts of Bellini: Papillary ducts; large collecting ducts in the nephrons

Dust cell: Phagocytic cell found in the alveoli of the lungs; also called an alveolar macrophage or an alveolar phagocyte

Decision Support System (DSS): Software and modelling methods used to aid management decision making under uncertainty.

Decision Support: Support for management decision making under uncertainty.

DEET: N,N-diethylmetatoluamide, an ingredient of insect repellents.

Defervescence: The reduction of a patient's abnormally elevated temperature into the normal range.

Deltamethrin: An insecticide.

Deltoideus:(G. deltoeides, shaped like the letter delta). The musculus deltoideus, shaped like an inverted delta.

Dentate:(L. dentatus, toothed). Notched muscles, e.g., the serrati.

Depression: An illness that involves the body, mood, and thoughts and that affects the way a person eats, sleeps, feels about himself or herself, and thinks about things.

Dermatitis: Inflammation of the skin, either due to direct contact with an irritating substance, or to an allergic reaction. Symptoms of dermatitis include redness, itching, and in some cases blistering.

Diaphragm:(G. diaphragma, a partition). Muscle diaphragma separating the thorax from the abdomen.

Diarrhea: A common condition that involves unusually frequent and liquid bowel movements. The opposite of constipation.

Digastricus:(G. di, two + gaster, belly). Denoting muscles with two fleshy parts separated by a tendinous intersection, e.g., musculus digastricus.

Dilatores:(ME. dilaten, to dilate or expand). Denoting a muscle that opens an orifice.

Dimension: Generally, a coordinate in any conceptual space, whereby a quantity or quality can be varied along a continuum or a discrete number of states

Diurnal: During the daytime.

Dizziness: Painless head discomfort with many possible causes including disturbances of vision, the brain, balance (vestibular) system of the inner ear, and gastrointestinal system. Dizziness is a medically indistinct term which laypersons use to describe a variety of conditions ranging from lightheadedness, unsteadiness to vertigo.

Drain: A device for removing fluid from a cavity or wound. A drain is typically a tube or wick. As a verb, to allow fluid to be released from a confined area.

Dorso-(L. dorsum, back). Muscles related to the dorsal surface of the body, e.g., latissimus dorsi muscle. Also any structure related specifically to the thorax.

Doxycycline: An antibiotic drug that can be used against malaria; by itself for prevention or in combination with either quinine or quinidine when used for treatment.

Driver: A parameter that is of central importance to a process or model, and which tends to "drive" other parameters. A factor that influences many other factors, but is itself less influenced.

Drug resistance: Drug resistance is the result of microbes changing in ways that reduce or eliminate the effectiveness of drugs, chemicals, or other agents to cure or prevent infections.

Dyspnea: Shallow, labored breathing.

E

Eccrine sweat gland: Sweat glands distributed over almost all the body

Elastic cartilage:A type of cartilage in which there are elastic fibers in the matrix

Elastic fiber:A type of fiber found in cartilage and connective tissue which gives the tissue elasticity

Elastin: Protein found in elastic fibers

Endocardium: Lining of the heart

Endocrine gland: Ductless gland; secretes hormones

Endocytosis: The process by which large particles are brought into cells

Endometrial glands: Glands found in the epithelial lining of the uterus

Endometrium: Lining of the uterus

Endomysium: Connective tissue covering a muscle fiber

Endoneurium: Connective tissue which surrounds individual nerve fibers and associated Schwann cells

Endoplasmic reticulum: Organelle within cells; two varieties: smooth and rough

Endosteum: Lining of bone

Endothelium: Simple squamous epithelium lining the heart, blood vessels, and lymphatic vessels

Enterochromaffin cells:APUD cells with granules which are seen with chromium and sliver salts

Eosin: Eosin is an acid stain which binds to and stains basic structures (or negatively charged structures)

Eosinophil: Granuloycte; granules of this type of white blood cell take up the dye eosin

Ependymal cells: Cells which line the central cavity of the spinal cord and brain ventricles

Epicardium: Outer covering of the heart

Epidermis: The outer layer of the skin composed of stratified squamous epithelium

Epineurium: Connective tissue sheeth which surrounds a nerve

Epithelioreticular cells: Star shaped cells in the thymus which form a framework for lymphoctes

Epithelium: Basic tissue type which covers and lines body cavities and surfaces

Erythrocyte: Red blood cell

Erythropoiesis: Development of erythrocytes

Erythropoietin: Hormone made by the kidney which stimulates red blood cell production

Exocrine gland: Glands that secrete onto body surfaces or into body cavities

Exocytosis: Process by which particles are moved from the cell to the exterior

Extracellular matrix: The material in the space which is outside of cells

Epi-(G. epi, upon). Denoting a muscle attached to another structure, e.g., dorsoepitrochlearis muscle.

Efficacy: The power or capacity to produce a desired effect.

Elimination: In the context of malaria, reducing all local transmission down to zero cases within a defined geographic location.

ELISA: Enzyme-linked immunosorbent assay. This laboratory test is now often used to determine whether mosquito salivary glands are positive for sporozoites.

Emarginate. Notched, with a shape seemingly cut from the margin.

Entire. Referring to a smoothly unbroken margin.

Epinotum. An older, alternative name for the propodeum, the first segment of the abdomen, which is fused to the rear part of the thorax.

Erect. Referring to a hair standing nearly to straight up from the body surface.

Excised. With a deep cut or notch.

Eye. Referring to the compound eye, composed of few to many separate ommatidia, or facets.

Enzyme: A protein (or protein-based molecule) that speeds up a chemical reaction in a living organism. An enzyme acts as catalyst for specific chemical reactions, converting a specific set of reactants (called substrates) into specific products. Without enzymes, life as we know it would not exist.

Erythromycin: Erythromycin is a common antibiotic for treating bacterial infection. Sold under many brand names, including EES, Erycin and Erythromia

Empirical Inconsistency: A practical (empirical) incompatibility or discrepancy between two or more conditions or statements about the observed world (comp. Logical Inconsistency).

Endemic: Where disease occurs on a consistent basis.

Endophagic: An endophagic mosquito is a mosquito that feeds indoors.

Endophilic: An endophilic mosquito is a mosquito that tends to inhabit/rest indoors. Endophilism facilitates the blocking of malaria transmission through application of residual insecticides to walls.

Epidemic: The occurrence of more cases of disease than expected in a given area or among a specific group of people over a particular period of time.

Epidemiology: The study of the distribution and determinants of health-related states or events in specified populations, and the application of this study to the control of health problems.

Epistropheus:(G. epistropheus, the pivot). Muscles relating to the second cervical vertebra.

Epitrochlearis:(L. epi, upon + trochlearis, block or pulley). Pertaining to muscles associated with the humeral epichondyle.

Eradication: In the context of malaria, reducing the number of malaria parasites that circulate in the natural world to zero.

Erythrocyte: A red blood cell.

Erythrocytic stage: A stage in the life cycle of the malaria parasite found in the red blood cells. Erythrocytic stage parasites cause the symptoms of malaria.

Etiology: The cause or origin of a disease or disorder; the study of the factors that cause disease and of the method of their introduction into the host.

Exoerythrocytic stage: A stage in the life cycle of the malaria parasite found in liver cells (hepatocytes). Exoerythrocytic stage parasites do not cause symptoms.

Exophagic: An exophagic mosquito is a mosquito that feeds outdoors.

Exophilic: An exophilic mosquito tends to inhabit/rest outdoors. Residual insecticides in buildings are less effective at controlling exophilic mosquitoes.

Extensor:(L. ex-tendre, to stretch out). A muscle that , upon contraction, tends to straighten a limb. The antagonist of a flexor muscle.

F

Facet. The ommatidium, a basic unit of the compound eye.

Falcate. Sickle-shaped.

Femur (plural: femora). The third segment of the leg away from the body, following the coxa and trochanter.

Fenestra. A translucent cutilar thin spot.

Filiform. Thread-like, as often seen in the antennal funiculus with the segments all of about the same size.

Flagellate. Whip-like.

Foramen. An opening or impressed pit.

Fossa plural: fossae). (A relatively large and deep pit, such as the antennal fossa on the head where the first antennal segment is inserted.

Fovea (plural: foveae). A deep depression with well marked sides.

Foveate. Having multiple foveae (deep pits with well marked sides).

Foveolate. Having multiple small, deep pits that are deeper and larger than punctures, giving a coarser appearance.

Frons. Area above the clypeus, approximately in the center of the front of head. The frontal triangle, which is roughly triangular in shape and demarcated by grooves, is often included in this area.

Frontal area. The frons.

Frontal carina. A pair of longitudinal ridges on the head found dorsally behind the clypeus and between the antennal sockets. They vary in length and may be short and simple, longer and extending back to occipital margin, are vestigial or absent.

Frontal clypeal suture. Suture fro ming the posterior margin of the clypeus.

Frontal triangle. The triangular shaped area usually found in the frontal area of head.

Funiculus (plural: funiculi). All of the antennal segment taken together, except for the basal segment, the scape.

Family history: The family structure and relationships within the family, including information about diseases in family members.

FDA: Food and Drug Administration.

Falciparum: See *Plasmodium*.

Fansidar: Brand name of sulfadoxine-pyrimethamine, a drug used against malaria. Its value has been compromised by the emergence of drug-resistant malaria parasites.

Fasicle. Bundle

Fenestrae. Pore or small opening

Fenestrated capillaries. Capillaries with pores

Fibroblast. Cell which secetes the fibers and ground substance of connective tissue

Fibrocartilage.A type of cartilage that has thick collagen fibers in the matrix

Fibrous astrocyte. Type of astrocyte more common in white matter

Fimbriae. Finger like extensions on the fallopian tube

Flagellum. Whiplike extension seen on some cells and bacteria for propulsion

Follicle.1. Structure within the ovary 2. Structure within thyroid gland 3. Portion of hair embedded in the skin

Formed elements. Red blood cells, white blood cells and platelets

Foot process. Pedicel; portion of a podocyte

Foreign body giant cell. Formed by the fusion of macrophages

Fundic glands. Type of gastric gland

Fusiform cell. Spindle shaped cell

Femoris.(L. femur, thigh). Pertaining to the femur or thigh.

Hassall's corpuscle. Distinctive structure seen in the medulla of the thymus

Haversian canal. Central canal in an osteon which contain blood vessels

Haversian system. Osteon; central canal and the surrounding rings

Hematopoiesis. Development of blood cells

Hematoxylin. Basic tissue stain which binds to and stains nucleic acids so the nucleus of a cell stains blue

Hemosiderin. Amber-gold pigment formed by the breakdown of hemoglobin

Henle's layer. Layer in the hair follicle

Henle's loop. Hairpin region of the nephron

Hensen's cells. Supporting cell type in the spiral organ of Corti

Hepatocyte. The primary cell of the liver parenchyma

Hering's canals. Small bile ducts which connect to portal canals

Herrings bodies. Granules within axons in the neurohypophysis

Histiocyte. Connective tissue macrophage

Histology.A branch of anatomy; microscopic anatomy

Hofbauer cell. Cell type in the placenta

Holocrine gland.A type of gland in which entire cells break apart to from the secretions of that gland

Horizontal cell.1. Retinal neuron 2. Horizontal cell of Cajal-cell of the cerebral cortex

Howship's lacunae. Hollow area underneath osteoclasts from bone resorption

Huxley's layer. Layer in the hair follicle

Hyaline cartilage.A type of cartilage with a glassy appearance

Hydroxyapatite. Mineral crystal of bone and teeth

Hair loss: Hair loss is the thinning of hair on the scalp. The medical term for hair loss is alopecia. Alopecia can be temporary or permanent.

Headache: A pain in the head with the pain being above the eyes or the ears, behind the head (occipital), or in the back of the upper neck. **Heart failure:** Inability of the heart to keep up with the demands on it and, specifically, failure of the heart to pump blood with normal efficiency

Hair. A seta.

Head. The foremost part of the body containing the antennae, eyes, and mandibles.

Helcium. The much reduced and specialized presclerites of abdominal segment 3 that form a complex articulation within the posterior foramen of the petiole.

Humerus (plural: humeri). The "shoulder", anterior corners of the pronotum (the first segment of the thorax.

Hypopygium. The last sternite (a lower plate) of the abdomen.

Hypostoma. The anteroventral region of the head; that area of cuticle just behind the buccal cavity and forming its posterior margin. Sometimes called gula.

Hypostomal teeth. One or more pairs of triangular to rounded teeth that project forward from the anterior margin of the hypostoma.

Hallucis.(L. hallux, great toe). The muscles and tendons associated with the first digit of the foot.

Halofantrine: A drug used against malaria in some countries, but not recommended by CDC.

Chloroquine and Body Tissues

Hematocrit: The amount of blood consisting of red blood cells, measured as a percentage.

Hematologic: Having to do with the blood.

Hemoglobin: The red, oxygen-carrying protein found in red blood cells.

Hemolysis: Destruction of red blood cells. Malaria causes hemolysis when the parasites rupture the red blood cells in which they have grown.

Hepatocytes: Liver cells.

Hepatomegaly: Enlarged liver.

Herbal: 1. An adjective, referring to herbs, as in an herbal tea.
2. A noun, usually reflecting the botanical or medicinal aspects of herbs;

Humero-(G. homos, shoulder). Pertaining to the bone of the arm and a muscles associated with it.

Hyo-(G. hyoeides, hyoid). Relating to the U-shaped hyoid bone and muscles associated with it.

Hyoideus. See Hyo- above.

Hyper-Coherent: When the degree of compatibility or internal consistency between parameters in a morphological model is very high, and many possible solutions or outcomes are obtained (opposite of hyper-constrained).

Hyper-Constrained: When the degree of compatibility or internal consistency between parameters in a morphological model is very low, and very few possible solutions or outcomes are obtained (opposite of hyper-coherent).

Hypnozoite: Dormant form of malaria parasites found in liver cells. Hypnozoites occur only with *Plasmodium vivax* and *P. ovale.* After sporozoites (inoculated by the mosquito) invade liver cells, some sporozoites develop into dormant forms (the hypnozoites), which do not cause any symptoms.

Hypoglycemia: Low blood glucose. Hypoglycemia can occur in malaria. In addition, treatment with quinine and quinidine stimulate insulin secretion, reducing blood glucose.

I

I band. Light band seen on striated muscle; isotropic band

Immunoblast.A lymphocyte which has been stimulated by an antigen

Inclusions. Non living particles seen within a cell

Interalveolar septum. The tissue between two pulmonary alveoli

Intercalated disc. Cross bands seen in cardiac muscle

Intercalated ducts. Ducts lined by a simple epithelium draining a secretory unit

Intercalated neurons. Neurons between sensory and motor neurons; interneurons

Intermembranous bone. Bone which forms from direct deposit, as opposed to from a cartilagenous model

Internal elastic lamina.In arteries and arterioles, the elastic fibers at the junction of the tunica intima and tunica media

Interneurons. Neurons between sensory and motor neurons; the vast majority of neurons are interneurons

Internuncial neurons. Neurons between sensory and motor neurons; interneurons

Interstitial cells of Cajal. Found between the layers of smooth muscle in the GI tract involved in motility

Interstitial cells of Leydig. Cells which produce and secrete testosterone found in the interstitium of the testis

Intestinal absorptive cell. Cell with a brush border for absorption of nutrients

Intestinal glands. Tubular glands in the small intestinal mucosa

Islet of Langerhans. Cellular clusters seen in the pancreas that have an endocrine function

Isotropic band. Light band seen on striated muscle; I band

Iliacus.(L. ilium, groin). A muscle of the groin.

Icterus: See jaundice.

Ilio-(L. ilium, groin). **Pertaining to a muscle of the groin and ilium.**

Immune system: A complex system that is responsible for distinguishing a person from everything foreign to him or her and for protecting his or her body against infections and foreign substances.

Immune system: The cells, tissues and organs that assist the body to resist infection and disease by producing antibodies and/or cells that inhibit the multiplication of the infectious agent.

Immune: Protected against infection, usually by the presence of antibodies.

Immunity: Protection generated by the body's immune system, in response to previous malaria attacks, resulting in ability to control or lessen a malaria attack.

Immunization: The process or procedure by which a subject (person, animal, or plant) is rendered immune, or resistant to a specific disease. This term is often used interchangeably with vaccination or inoculation, although the act of inoculation does not always result in immunity.

Imported malaria: Malaria acquired outside a specific geographic area.

Inconsistency: When two statements or conditions are logically or empirically incompatible or contradictory.

Incubation period: The interval of time between infection by a microorganism and the onset of the illness or the first symptoms of the illness. In malaria, the incubation is between the mosquito bite and the first symptoms. Incubation periods range from 7 to 40 days, depending on species.

Indicis.(L. index, one that points). The forefinger or pointer.

Indigenous malaria: Mosquito-borne transmission of malaria in a geographic area where malaria occurs regularly.

Indoor residual spraying (IRS): Treatment of houses where people spend night-time hours, by spraying insecticides that have residual efficacy (i.e., that continue to affect mosquitoes for several months). Residual insecticide spraying aims to kills mosquitoes when they come to rest on the walls, usually after a blood meal.

Induced malaria: Malaria acquired through artificial means (e.g. blood transfusion, shared needles or syringes, or malariotherapy).

Infant: A young baby, from birth to 12 months of age.

Infection: The invasion and multiplication of microorganisms such as bacteria, viruses, and parasites that are not normally present within the body.

Infection: The invasion of an organism by a pathogen such as bacteria, viruses, or parasites. Some, but not all, infections lead to disease.

Inferior. In a lower anatomical position.

Inferior.(L. inferior, lower). Lower, caudal.

Influence diagram: In general, a qualitative model of a system, which depicts influence relationships between different elements or aspects of the system, shows the direction of such influences and (usually, but not always) allows for feedback loops or circular causality.

Infra-(L. infra, below) Pertaining to a position below a named structure, e.g., infraspinatus.

Inter.(L. inter, between). Between or among.

Internal.(L. internus, interior). Deep or away from the surface.

Introduced malaria: Mosquito-borne transmission of malaria from an imported case in a geographic area where malaria does not occur regularly.

Ischio-(G. ischion, hip) Pertaining to the ischium.

Itching: An uncomfortable sensation in the skin that feels as if something is crawling on the skin and makes the person want to scratch the affected area. Itching is medically known as pruritis; something that is itchy is pruritic.

J

Jaundice: Yellow discoloration of skin and eyes due to elevated blood levels of bilirubin.

Joint. A segment, such as a joint of the antenna.

Junctional complex. Intercellular attachment

Juxtaglomerular cells. Portion of the juxtaglomerular apparatus which secretes renin

Juxtamedullary nephron. Nephron that has its glomerulus next to the base of a renal pyramid

K

Karyokinesis. Nuclear division

Keratin. Protein found in epidermis, hair and nails

Keratinocyte. Cell found in the epidermis of the skin which produces keratin

Keratohyaline granules. Granules seen in the stratum granulosum

Killer T cell. Type of T lymphoctye; cytotoxic T cell

Kinocilium. Long cilia

Kohn's pores. Channels between adjacent alveoli

Kupffer cell. Hepatic macrophage

Kidney: One of a pair of organs located in the right and left side of the abdomen. The kidneys remove waste products from the blood and produce urine.

Knowlesi: See *Plasmodium*

L

Labial palps. A pair of jointed appendages (sensory palps) that arise anterolaterally from the labium and having a maximum of 4 segments.

Labium. The second maxilla, which forms a lower lip beneath the maxillae.

Labrum. A broad lobe suspended from the clypeus above the mouth and forming and upper lip.

Lamella. A thin plate-like process.

Lanuginous. Down-like or wooly.

Leg segments. An appendage, used for locomotion or support and consisting of a basal coxa that articulates from the alitrunk, followed in order by a small trochanter, a long femur (often somewhat stout), a tibia, and a tarsus, which consists of five small segments and terminating in a pair of claws apically.

Lobiform. Lobe-shaped.

Laboratory: A place for doing tests and research procedures, and for preparing chemicals and some medications. Also known as lab.

Lariam: Brand name of mefloquine, a drug used against malaria for both prevention and treatment.

Larvae: An immature stage of a developing mosquito.Â Mosquito larvae are wingless and develop in water.

Lateral.(L. lateralis, lateral). To the right or left of the axial line, to the outside, away from the midline.

Latissimo-(L. latus, broad). A term applied to some broad flat muscles, e.g., latissimus dorsi.

Leukocyte: White blood cell.

Leukocytosis: Increase in total white blood cell count.

Leukopenia: Decrease in total white blood cell count.

Levator.(L. levare, to lift). One of several muscles whose function is to lift the structure to which it is attached, e.g., levator palpebrae superiorus.

Linguae.(L. lingua, tongue). Pertaining to, or toward, the tongue.

Linkage (Linkage structure): Concerns how parameters in a Morphological Field are linked, i.e. which parameters constrain each other, and which do not.

Liver disease: Liver disease refers to any disorder of the liver. The liver is a large organ in the upper right abdomen that aids in digestion and removes waste products from the blood.

Lupus: A chronic inflammatory disease that is caused by autoimmunity. Patients with lupus have in their blood unusual antibodies that are targeted against their own body tissues.

Liver: The largest solid organ in the body, situated in the upper part of the abdomen on the right side.

Logical Inconsistency (Analytic Contradiction): A logical incompatibility or contradiction between two or more statements. A "contradiction in terms" (comp. Empirical Inconsistency) Lacteals

Lymphatic capillaries that are found in the villi of the small intestine

Lactotrops. Acidophilic cells in the adenohypophysis which secrete prolactin

Lacunae. Small space or cavity

Lamella. Layer

Lamina propria. Connective tissue layer underneath epithelium

Lamina vitrea. The inner layer of the choroid; also called Bruch's membrane

Langerhans cells. Star shaped macrophages found in the epidermis; antigen presenting cells

Leukocytes. White blood cells. Specifically: neutrophils, lymphocytes, monocytes, eosinophils, and basophils

Leydig cells. Cells which produce and secrete testosterone found in the interstitium of the testis

Lieberkühn crypts. Glands found in the epithelium of the small intestine

Lipocyte. Cell which stores fat (often used specifically for fat storing cell in liver)

Lipofuscin. Amber or brown pigment sometimes found in older cells

Liquor folliculi. The fluid in the antrum of an ovarian follicle

Littoral cells. Lining cells seen in the spleen, lymphatic sinuses and bone marrow

Loop of Henle. Hair pin shaped region of the nephron

Luschka's ducts. Accessory cystic duct

Lymphatic follicles. Concentrated spherical aggregates of lymphatic tissue which is found in the gastrointestinal, respiratory and genitourinary systems

Lymphatic nodule. Concentrated aggregate of lymphatic tissue; found in GI, respiratory and genitourinary systems

Lymphoblast. Immature lymphocyte

Lymphocyte. Agranular leukocyte

Lysosome. Membrane bound organelle; suicide sac

Longissimus.(L. longus, long). A name given to certain long muscles, e.g., longissimus capitis.

Lumborum.(L. lumbus, a loin) Pertaining to the back and sides between the pelvis and ribs.

Lumbricales.(L. lumbricus, an earthworm). Muscles resembling earthworms, e.g. the lumbricals.

Lymphocyte: Leukocyte with a large round nucleus and usually a small cytoplasm. Specialized types of lymphocytes have enlarged cytoplasms and produce antibodies. Other specialized lymphocytes are important in cellular immune responses.

M

M line. Center of the H band in a sarcomere

Macrophage. Phagocytic cell derived from monocytes

Macula adherens. Type of cell junction; important juction within epithelial tissue; desmosome

Macula densa. Specialized cells in the distal convoluted tubule; part of the juxtaglomerular apparatus

Macula pellucid. Stigma; site on the surface of the ovary where oocyte rupture occurs

Mall's space. Region in liver where lymph is formed

Malpighian corpuscle.1. Renal corpuscle 2. Splenic nodule

MALT. Mucosal associated lymphatic tissue

Martinotti cell. Type of nerve cell found in the cerebral cortex

Mast cells. Connective tissue cell with granules which contain heparin and histamine

Medulla. Inner portion of organ

Megakaryocyte. Giant cell found in the bone marrow; fragments form platelets

Meiosis. Process of nuclear division during the generation of sex cell which cuts the number of chromosomes in half

Meissner's corpuscle. Tactile receptors sensitive to light touch found in the dermis

Meissner's plexus. Submucosal plexus of the gastrointestinal tract

Melanin. Dark pigment formed by melanocytes

Melanocyte. Cells in the skin at the epidermal/dermal junction which produce melanin

Membrane bone. Bone which forms from direct deposit, as opposed to from a cartilagenous model

Memory cell. Lymphocyte that has been exposed to a specific antigen so that when re-exposed to that antigen it can recognize the antigen and rapidly divide

Merkel cell. Tactile receptor in the skin

Mesenchyme. Embryonic connective tissue

Mesangial cells. Cell type seen in the glomerulus; interstitial cells

Mesothelium. Type of epithelium which lines some internal body cavities

Metamyelocyte. Cell type in granulopoiesis

Metarteriole. Vessel which is in between arteriole and capillary

Microglia. Type of neuroglia; CNS macrophages

Microvilli. Projections on the apical surface of some epithelial cells which increase the surface area for absorpiton

Mitochondria. Cellular organelles which generates ATP; powerhouse of the cell

Mitosis. Nuclear division seen with cell division

Mixed glands. Glands which are composed of both serous cells and mucous cells

Monocyte. Agranular white blood cell; largest white blood cell

Mucosa. Mucous membrane; lining of passageways

Mucos connective tissue. Type of mesenchyme

Mucous neck cell.A type of mucous secreting cell found in the stomach

Mueller cell. Supporting cell in the retina

Multipolar cell. Cell with many processes

Muscle fiber. Muscle cell

Myelin. Fatty sheeth surrounding nerve cell processes

Myelocyte. Cell type seen in granulopoiesis

Myeloid. Cell line in the bone marrow

Myenteric plexus. Plexus that is between the two layers of external muscle in the GI tract; Auerbach's plexus

Myoepithelial cells. Embryologically from ectoderm; contactile cells

Myofibril. Longitudinal unit within a muscle fiber

Myosin. Contractile protein that is very prevalent in muscle

Macrochaetae. Large, standing, setae, often barbulate (barbs are often small and high magnification is needed to veiw them); sometimes referred to as pilosity. Common in such genera as *Paratrechina*.

Mandibles. The first pair of jaws, usually with teeth. These appendages are used by ants to manipulate their environment and vary in size, shape, and dentition.

Macrogametocyte: The female form of the gametocyte.

Macrolide: One in a class of antibiotics that includes Biaxin, Clarithromycin, Ery-Tab, and Erythromycin.

Magnesium: A mineral involved in many processes in the body including nerve signaling, the building of healthy bones, and normal muscle contraction.

Malaria: An infectious disease caused by protozoan parasites from the Plasmodium family that can be transmitted by the sting of the Anopheles mosquito or by a contaminated needle or transfusion. Falciparum malaria is the most deadly type.

Malariae: See *Plasmodium*.

Malarone: Brand name of atovaquone-proguanil, a drug used against malaria for both prevention and treatment.

Mandibulo-(L. mandere, to chew). Pertaining to a muscle arising from the mandible.

Manus.(L. manus, hand). Pertaining to the muscles of the hand.

Masseter.(G. maseter, masticator). A large masticatory muscle of the jaw.

Mastoideus.(G. mastos, breast + eidos, resemblance). Resembling a mamma or a breast- shaped structure.

Maxilla (plural: maxillae). The second pair of jaws, usually folded beneath the first pair of jaws, the mandibles.

Maxillary palps. The pair of jointed sensory appendages (palps) that arise from the maxillae with a maximum of 6 segments.

Median. The middle.

Mesopleuron (Plural-Mesopleura). The middle and largest pleuron of the thorax, sometimes divided by a transverse groove in an upper area, the anepisternum, and a lower area, the katepisternum.

Mesonotum. The tergite of the mesothorax (the second or middle part of the thorax).

Mesosoma. The middle of the three major body parts, also called the alitrunk.

Metanotal groove. A transverse groove or impression separating the mesonotum and propodeum.

Metanotum. The tergite of the metathorax (the third or last segment of the thorax).

Metasternal process. A paired cuticular projection of the posteroventral alitrunk sometimes present. When present, found astride the ventral midline, anterior to the apex of the cavity that the petiole articulates and near the level of the anterior margins of the metacoxal cavities.

Metathorax. See thorax.

Metatibia. Tibial segment of the metathorax (third or hind part of thorax).

Metatibial gland. A gland thought to be and exocrine gland, found ventrally on the metatibia posterior to the tibial spur.

Medial.(L. medialis, middle). Relating to muscle nearer to the median or midsagittal plane.

Medical history: In clinical medicine, the patient's past and present which may contain clues bearing on their health past, present, and future.

Mefloquine: A drug used against malaria for both prevention and treatment.

Mentalis.(L. mentum, chin). Relating to the muscles of the chin, e.g., musculus mentalis.

Mento-(L. mentum, chin). See Mentalis.

Merozoite: A daughter cell formed by asexual development in the life cycle of malaria parasites. Liver-stage and blood-stage malaria parasites develop into schizonts which contain many merozoites.

 Mess: (See: Social Mess)

Metacarpo-(G. meta, after + carpus, wrist). Pertaining to the bones adjacent to the wrist.

Chloroquine and Body Tissues

Microgametocyte: The male form of the gametocyte.

Model: A simplified, schematic representation of a system or phenomenon that accounts for its known or inferred properties and may be used for further study of its characteristics. Scientific models usually delineate the system's or phenomenon's variables and relate such variables to one another. modeling the relations can be logical (e.g. consistency) or pertain merely to influence (influence diagram).

Molecular methods: Laboratory techniques that are based on identification and characterization of certain molecules and gene sequences of a pathogen's genetic makeup.

Monocyte: Leukocyte with a large, usually kidney-shaped nucleus. Within tissues, monocytes develop into macrophages which ingest bacteria, dead cells, and other debris.

Morphological Analysis: The study of form or structure by identifying the multiple dimensions comprising any system, e.g. an organism, an organisation, a conceptual system or any entity taken as a whole. Employed in e.g. Zoology, Botany, Geology and Linguistics. (See General Morphological Analysis)

Morphological Field: The field of constructed dimensions or parameters which is the basis for a morphological model.

Morphological Model: A morphological field with its parameters assessed and linked through a Cross-Consistency Assessment (CCA).

Morphology: The study of form or structure; how parts of a system *conform* to create a whole or Gestalt.

Mouth: The upper opening of the digestive tract, beginning with the lips and containing the teeth, gums, and tongue. Foodstuffs are broken down mechanically in the mouth by chewing and saliva is added as a lubricant.

Multi-Driver Inputs: Using multiple drivers as input to a morphological model in order to determine numerous possible outputs or results. (See Driver)

Muscle: Muscle is the tissue of the body which primarily functions as a source of power.

Musculus.(L. mus, mouse). A muscle.

Myo-(G. mys, a muscle). Relating to a muscle.

Mytiformis.(G. mytilos, mussel + forma, shape). Shaped like the shellfish, e.g., musculus mytiformis.

N

Nail bed. Structure that the nail plate rests on

Natural killer cell. Type of lymphocyte; NK cell

Nephron. The functional unit of the kidney which is composed of a glomerulus and a uriniferous tubule

Neurofilaments. Intermediate fibers of neurons

Neuroglia. Supporting cells of the central nervous system

Neurolemma. Outermost covering of nerve fiber; also spelled neurilemma

Neuron. Nerve cell

Neurosecretory cell. Neuron which secretes a hormone

Neutrophil. Type of white blood cell; granulocyte in which the granules show no particicular attraction for either acidic or basic dyes

Nissl bodies. Distinctive rough endoplasmic reticulum and ribosomes seen in neurons

Node of Ranvier. Area between two Schwann cells which is not covered by myelin

Nonlamellar bone. Immature bone; woven bone

Normoblast.**Cell seen in erythropoiesis which has a compact nucleus**

Nucleolus.Region in the nucleus of a cell where ribosomal RNA production occurs

Nucleus. Part of the cell which contains the genetic information

Naris(L. naris, nostril). Pertaining to muscles associated with the nostril.

Nasalis(L. nasus, nose). Pertaining to the nose.

Nuchae(F. nuque, back of the neck). Muscles associated with the back of the neck.

Nausea: Stomach queasiness, the urge to vomit. Nausea can be brought on by many causes, including systemic illnesses (such as influenza), medications, pain, and inner ear disease.

Node. A rounded, knob-like structure as in the petiolar node, the upper rounded part of the petiole.

Nuchal collar. A ridge on the head found posteriorly and separating the dorsal and lateral surfaces from the occipital surface.

Normative Inconsistency (Normative Constraint): An incompatibility or discrepancy between two or more conditions based on social norms, ethics and standards.

Nursing: 1) Profession concerned with the provision of services essential to the maintenance and restoration of health by attending the needs of sick persons. 2) Feeding a infant at the breast.

O

Occipital lobes. The rear corners of the head.

Occipital margin. The transverse posterior margin of the head in full-face view; actually this term is incorrect morphologically, as the occiput proper usually begins behind this level, but the name is acceptable for most purposes.

Occiput. Referring to the rearmost part of the head.

Ocellus (plural: ocelli). One of the simple, bead shaped eyes found in the rear central part of the head.

Ommatidium (plural: ommatidia). A facet, or unit, of the compound eye.

Occipitalis.(L. ob, before or against + caput, head). Pertaining to muscles attached to the occipital bone.

Odontoblast. Cells which produce dentin in the tooth pulp

Olfactory mucosa. Mucosa lining parts of the nasal cavity

Oligodendrocyte. Glial cell in the CNS which wraps around axons to form myelin sheaths

Oocyte. Developing female gamete; immature ovum

Optic disc. The area of the retina that the optic nerve leaves from; responsible for the blind spot

Ora serrata. Junction between the ciliary body and the retina

Organ of Corti. Part of the cochlea; houses the auditory sensory receptors

Omo.(L. omo, shoulder). Pertaining to muscle attached to the scapula.

Oocyst: A stage in the life cyle of malaria parasites, oocysts are rounded structures located in the outer wall of the stomach of mosquitoes.

Opponens.(L. opponere, to place against). A name given to several adductor muscles of the fingers and toes.

Organelle. Specialized intracellular structure

Osteoblast. Bone forming cell

Osteoclast. Multinucleated cell which breaks done bone matrix

Osteocyte. Mature bone cell

Osteoid. Bone matrix which is unmineralized

Osteon. Structural unit in mature bone consisting of concentric layers of bone lamellae around the central canal

Ova. Mature female gamete

Oxyntic cell. Also called a parietal cell. Cell found in the stomach which produces hydrochloric acid and intrinsic factor

Oxyphilic cell. One of the two main cell types found in the parathyroid gland

Oxytalan fibers. Fibers in the periodontal ligament

Obturator.(L. obturare, to occlude). Pertaining to muscles associated with the obturator membrane, which closes the obturator foramen.

Oris.(L. oris, mouth). Relating to the entrance to the digestive tube, or mouth.

Os.(L. os, bone) a bone

Ovale: See *Plasmodium.*

P

Pacinian corpuscle. Mechanoreceptor for pressure

Pampiniform plexus. Venous plexus found in the reproductive system

Paneth cells. Cells with prominent granules found in the deepest part of an intestinal gland

Papillary layer. Superficial layer of the dermis

Parafollicular cells. Cell type in a thyroid follicle which secretes calcitonin; also called a C cells

Parenchyma. The functional portion of an organ

Parakeratinized epithelium. Keratinized epithelium where the cells still have their nuclei

Parietal cell. Also called a oxyntic cell. Found in the stomach; produces HCl and intrinsic factor

Pars convolute. Distal convoluted tubule

Pars distalis. Anterior lobe of the pituitary

Pars intermedia. Intermediate lobe of pituitary

Pars nervosa. Posterior lobe of pituitary

Pars recta. Proximal straight tubule in the kidney

Pars tuberalis. Portion of adenohypophysis around infundibuluar stem

Pedicel. Foot process of a podocyte

Peg cells. Non-ciliated secretory cells found in the oviduct

Periarterial lymphatic sheath.PALS; cluster of lymphoctes surrounding a central artery of the spleen

Perichondrium. Connective tissue covering which surrounds cartilage

Pericyte. An undifferentiated cell seen in association with some capillaries

Perikaryon. The cell body of a nerve cell

Perimetrium. Covering of the uterus

Perimysium. Connective tissue sheath surrounding muscle fascicles

Perineurium. Connective tissue sheath surrounding nerve fibers

Periodontium. Supporting tissue of the teeth

Periosteum. Connective tissue covering of bone

Peyer's patches. Lymphoid nodules seen in the lamina propria of the large intestine and appendix

Phagocytosis. Form of endocytosis; "cell eating"

Phalangeal cells. Supporting cells of the spiral organ

Pillar cells. Cell type found in the organ of Corti

Pinocytosis.A form of endoctyosis in which fluids enter the cell; 'cell drinking'

Pituicyte. Cell type found in the neurohypophysis

Plasma cell. Cell derived from B lymphoctyes which secretes antibodies

Plasma membrane. The cell membrane

Plasmalemma. The cell membrane

Platelet. Cell fragment in blood which is involved in clotting

Pleomorphic. Having a variety of shapes and sizes

Pneumocyte. Cell of the pulmonary alveoli

Podocytes. Octopus shaped cells which surround glomerular capillaries

Polychromatophilic erythroblast. Immature cell in the development of the red blood cell

Polychromatophilic erythrocyte. Reticulocyte

Polymorph.PMN; neutrophil

Polymorphonuclear leukocyte.PMN; neutrophil

Pores of Kohn. Channels between adjacent alveoli

Portal triad. Seen in the liver; branch of the hepatic artery, hepatic portal vein, and bile duct

Predentin. Matrix of dentin

PP cells.Cells of the pancreas which secrete pancreatic polypeptide

Preosteoblast. Osteoprogenitor cell; cell which will differentiate into osteoblast

Presynaptic membrane. Region of a nerve cell abutting the synaptic cleft

Primary follicle. Follicular stage where the primary oocyte is surrounded by cuboidal cells

Primary nodule. Aggregation of small lymphocytes

Primordial follicle. Primitive follicle

Principal cell.1. Parathyroid cell which secretes parathyroid hormone 2. Cell type in the thyroid; follicular cells

Proerythroblast. Immature cell in the development of the red blood cell

Promyelocyte. Primitive cell in granulopoiesis

Prostatic concretions. Corpora amylaceae; eosinophilic bodies seen in the prostate

Proximal convoluted tubule.PCT, part of the nephron

Psammoma body. Concentric whorls seen in choroid plexus, meninges, pineal gland, and some tumors

Pseudopod. Non permanent project of the cytoplasm of a cell

Pseudostratified epithelium.A type of epithelium where all cells touch the basement membrane yet has the appearance of being stratified

Pseudounipolar neuron. Unipolar neuron

Purkinje cells. Cell type in the cerebellum

Purkinje fibers. Specialized cardiac muscle fibers inolved in the transmission of the impulse from the atrioventricular node to the ventricles

Pyramidal cells. Neurons in the cerebral cortex with a cell body shaped like a pyramid

Pain: An unpleasant sensation that can range from mild, localized discomfort to agony. Pain has both physical and emotional components.

Palato-(L. palatum, palate). Relating to the hard or soft palate.

Palmaris.(L. palma, palm of the hand). Pertaining to muscles of the forearm, wihich may insert into the palmar aponeurosis.

Palpebrae.(L. palpebra, eyelid). The eyelid.

Panniculus.(L. pannus, cloth). Pertaining to a thin sheet of dermal muscle.

Paramere. Two lateral processes sheathing the male aedeagus.

Pectinate. Comb-like, such as some structures including the tibial spurs.

Pedicel. Either the "waist" (petiole and postpetiole combined) or the the second segment of the antenna from the base outward. When referring to the segment(s) found between the alitrunk and gaster, waist is the preferred term.

Pedunculate. Stalk-like, or set on a stalk or peduncle.

Petiole. The first, and sometimes the only, segment of the waist, found between the propodeum and the gaster.

Phragmotic. Sharply truncated as seen in the overall front of the head of some stem dwelling Camponotus, subgenus Coloboposis species.

Piligerous. Bearing a hair.

Pilosity. The longer and stouter hairs that stand above the shorter and usually finer hairs that make up the pubescence. Sometimes referred to as macrochaetae, especially if barbulate.

Pleurite/pleuron. The lateral sclerites of the thorax proper, excluding the propodeum (which is actually the first segment of the abdomen, but fused to the thorax).

Plumose. Referring to hairs that are multiply branched and feather-like in appearance.

Postpetiole. The second segment of the waist, some ants do not have a postpetiole.

Presclerite. A distinctly differentiated anterior section of an abdominal sclerite and separated from the remainder of the sclerite by a ridge, constriction, or both.

Pretarsal claws. A pair of claws on the pretarsal (apical) tarsal segment of the leg.

Pretarsus. Terminal segment of the foot, with a pair of claws and usually an arolium, or central pad.

Pronotum. The tergite of the prothorax (the first segment of the thorax).

Propodeal spine. Spine present on ants and articulating from the propodeum.

Propodeum. The first abdominal segment that is fused to the rear of the thorax, also called the epinotum.

Promesonotal suture. The transverse suture on the dorsum of the alitrunk separating the pronotum from the mesonotum.

Promesonotum. The fused pronotum and mesonotum taken together.

Prothorax. See thorax.

Proximal. Closest with reference to the body.

Pruinose. With a frosted or slightly dusted appearance.

Psammophore. Basket-like grouping of long, curved hairs found beneath the head of some ants.

Pubescence. Very short, fine hairs, usually forming a second layer beneath the pilosity.

Punctate. Having fine punctures like pinpricks.

Punctures. Small, pinpoint impressions in the exoskeleton.

Pygidium. The last complete tergite (upper plate) of the abdomen.

Parameter space: A set of mutually linked parameters making up the Morphological Field.

Parameter Values: (see also "Conditions"): The different states or values a parameter can take on; the parameter's value range. **"Problem"**: Use by Russel Ackoff ("Redesigning the Future", 1974) to denote a well-defined issue where the parameters and the mutual relationships between parameters are known, but where there is no single, unequivocal solution.

Parameter: One of a set of measurable factors that defines a system and determines its behaviour, and which can be varied in an experiment.

Parasite: A plant or an animal organism that lives in or on another and takes its nourishment from that other organism. Parasitic diseases include infections that are due to protozoa, helminths, or arthropods. For example, malaria is caused by Plasmodium, a parasitic protozoa.

Parasite: Any organism that lives in or on another organism without benefiting the host organism; commonly refers to pathogens, most commonly in reference to protozoans and helminths.

Parasitemia: The presence of parasites in the blood. The term can also be used to express the quantity of parasites in the blood (e.g., "a parasitemia of 2%").

Paroxysm: A sudden attack or increase in intensity of a symptom, usually occurring in intervals.

Pathogen: Bacteria, viruses, parasites or fungi can cause disease.

Pectineus.(L. pecten, a comb). Pertaining to the os pubis or any ridged structure. A muscle.

Pectoro-(L.pectus, pector-, chest). Pertaining to the muscles of the chest wall.

Chloroquine and Body Tissues

Pedis.(L. pes, foot). Refering to the foot.

Penis.(L. penis, tail) The male reproductive organ.

Permethrin: A pyrethroid insecticide.

Peroneus.(G. perone, brooch or fibula). Pertaining to several muscles on the lateral or fibular side of the leg.

Phagocyte: A type of white blood cell that can engulf and destroy foreign organisms, cells and particles. Phagocytes are an important part of the immune system.

Phalangei.(F., G., L. phalanx, a formation of Roman soldiers). Pertaining to the bones of the fingers.

Pharmacist: A professional who fills prescriptions and, in the case of a compounding pharmacist, makes them. Pharmacists are very familiar with medication ingredients, interactions, and cautions.

Pharyngeus.(G. pharynx, throat). Pertaining to the pharynx.

Piriformis.(L. pirum, pear + forma, shaped). Pear-shaped.

Pisiform.(L. pisum, pea + forma). Pea-shaped or pea sized.

Plantaris.(L. plantaris, sole of the foot) Pertaining to a muscle of the foot, musculus plantaris.

Plasmodium: The genus of the parasite that causes malaria. The genus includes many species

Platelets: Small, irregularly-shaped bodies in the blood that contain granules. These cells are important components of the blood coagulation (clotting) system.

Platysma.(G. platys, flat or broad). A broad flat dermal muscle of the thorax and neck.

Poison control center: A special information center set up to inform people about how to respond to potential poisoning. These centers maintain databases of poisons and appropriate emergency treatment. Local poison control centers should be listed with other community-service numbers in the front of the telephone book, and they can also be reached immediately through any telephone operator.

Poison: Any substance that can cause severe organ damage or death if ingested, breathed in, or absorbed through the skin. Many substances that normally cause no problems, including water and most vitamins, can be poisonous if taken in excessive quantity. Poison treatment depends on the 'substance.

Pollicis.(L. pollex, thumb). Relating to the thumb.

Polymorphic: Literally meaning having more than one form. In terms of genes it means that there are several variants (alleles) of a particular gene that occur simultaneously in a population.

Popliteus.(L. poples, the ham of the knee). Pertaining to a muscle of the popliteal space.

Porphyria: One of a variety of hereditary diseases that are characterized by abnormalities in the reactions needed for the production of heme, an essential substance for the body, resulting in increased formation and excretion of chemicals called porphyrins.

Potassium: The major positive ion (cation) found inside cells

Pregnancy: The state of carrying a developing embryo or fetus within the female body. This condition can be indicated by positive results on an over-the-counter urine test, and confirmed through a blood test, ultrasound, detection of fetal heartbeat, or an X-ray.

Pregnant: The state of carrying a developing fetus within the body.

Prescription: A physician's order for the preparation and administration of a drug or device for a patient. A prescription has several parts.

Presumptive treatment: Treatment of clinically suspected cases without, or prior to, results from confirmatory laboratory tests.

Primaquine: A drug used against malaria for the prevention of *P. vivax* or for the eradication of the hypnozoites of *P. vivax* and *P. ovale*.

Problem space: The totality of the possible configurations obtained in a Morphological Field (see Solution space).

Problem Structuring Methods: A family of methods that apply modelling approaches to address messy or wicked problems faced by managers of organizations. These methods seek to alleviate or improve situations characterised by uncertainty, conflict and complexity.

Procerus.(L. procerus, long or stretched-out). A muscle of the nose.

Proguanil: A drug used against malaria. It is found in the combination atovaquone-proguanil which can be used for both prevention and treatment.

Pronator.(L. pronare, to bend forward). A muscle that, on contraction, rotates the hand so that the palm of the hand faces backward when the arm is in the anatomical position.

Prophylaxis: See "chemoprophylaxis."

Protozoan: Single-celled organism that can perform all necessary functions of metabolism and reproduction. Some protozoa are free-living, while others, including malaria parasites, parasitize other organisms for their nutrients and life cycle.

Psoas.(G. psoa, muscle of the loin). Pertaining to muscles in the lumbosacral region, the "tenderloin".

Psoriasis: A reddish, scaly rash often located over the surfaces of the elbows, knees, scalp, and around or in the ears, navel, genitals or buttocks.

Pterygoideus.(G. pteryx, or pteryg-, wing + eidos, resemblance). Wing-shaped. Applied to muscles associated with the pterygoid processes of the sphenoid bone.

Pubo-(L. pubes, genitalis). Pertaing to muscles attaching to the os pubis.

Pyramidalis.(G. pyramis, pyramid). Applied to muscles having, more or less, pyramidal shape.

Pyrethroid: A class of insecticides derived from the natural pyrethrins.

Q

Quadratus.(L. quadratus, square). More or less square-shaped muscles.

Quadriceps.(L. quadi-, four + caput, head). A name given to a muscle having four heads, e.g., quadriceps femoris.

Quinine: A drug used against malaria, obtained from the bark of the cinchona tree. Quinine is used for treatment but not prevention of malaria.

Quinti.(L. quintus, fifth). Fifth, as in the fifth digit.

R

Rabies: A potentially fatal viral infection that attacks the central nervous system. Rabies is carried by wild animals (particularly bats and raccoons) and finds its way to humans by many routes.

Radical cure: (also: radical treatment) Complete elimination of malaria parasites from the body; the term applies specifically to elimination of dormant liver stage parasites (hypnozoites) found in *Plasmodium vivax* and *P. ovale*.

Radical treatment: See radical cure.

Ranvier's node. Area between two Schwann cells which is not covered by myelin

Red blood cell. Erythrocyte

Red fiber. Type of muscle fiber which make up slow twitch motor units

Red pulp. Tissue in the spleen composed of splenic sinuses and splenic cords

Reinke crystals. Crystals seen in the interstitial cells of Leydig

Renal columns.Kidney tissue which is between the pyramids

Renal corpuscle. Glomerulus and Bowman's capsule

Residual body. Accumulation of indigestable matter within a cell

Respiratory bronchiole. First portion of the respiratory tract where gas exchange actually occurs

Rete ovarii. Fetal remnants within the ovary

Rete testis. Tubules within the testis

Rete peg. Regions in the skin where the stratum germinativum projects downward into the dermis

Reticular. Network

Reticular fiber. Type of fiber made of collagen

Reticular layer. Deeper region within the dermis

Reticuloctye. Immature erythrocyte (RBC); also called polychromatophilic erythrocyte

Reticuloendothelial system. Component of the immune system consisting of the phagocytic cells within the reticular connective tissue

Retina. The sensory tunic of the eye

Recrudescence: A repeated attack of malaria due to the survival of malaria parasites in red blood cells.

Rectalis.(L. rectus, straight). Pertaining to muscles associated with the distal segment of the large intestine.

Red blood cells: The blood cells that carry oxygen. Red cells contain hemoglobin and it is the hemoglobin which permits them to transport oxygen (and carbon dioxide). Hemoglobin, aside from being a transport molecule, is a pigment. It gives the cells their red color (and their name).

Reflex: An involuntary reaction. For example, the corneal reflex is the blink that occurs upon irritation of the eye.

Chloroquine and Body Tissues

Relapse: Recurrence of disease after it has been apparently cured. In malaria, true relapses are caused by reactivation of dormant liver stage parasites (hypnozoites) found in *Plasmodium vivax* and *P. ovale.*

Relapse: The return of signs and symptoms of a disease after a remission.

Replete. Swollen with liquid food.

Reticulate. Being covered with a network of carinae, striae, or rugae.

Reticulate-punctate. Being covered with a network of carinae, striae, or rugae with punctures in the interspaces.

Ruga (plural: rugae). A wrinkle.

Rugoreticulate. A network or grid formed by rugae.

Rugose. Having multiple wrinkles, usually running parallel.

Rugula (plural: rugulae). Small wrinkle.

Rugulose. Having multiple small wrinkles, usually running parallel.

Residual insecticide spraying: See indoor residual spraying.

Resistance: The ability of an organism to develop ways to be impervious to specific threats to their existence. The malaria parasite has developed strains that are resistant to drugs such as chloroquine. The *Anopheles* mosquito has developed strains that are resistant to DDT and other insecticides.

Rhombo-(G. rhombos, a rhomb). Resembling a rhomb, an oblique parallelogram of unequal sides. Relating to two superficial muscles of the back.

Ribosome. Cytoplasmic organelle which produces proteins

RNA. Ribonucleic acid

Rod cell. Type of photoreceptors in the retina

Rokitansky-Aschoff sinuses. Diverticula seen in the mucosa of the gallbladder

Rough endoplasmic reticulum. Endoplasmic reticulum which is studded with ribosomes

Ruffini's corpuscle. Tactile receptor responsive to continuous pressure

Ruffled border. Plasma membrane foldings on an osteoclast

Radio-(L. radius, ray). Pertaining to muscles associated with the radius of the forearm.

Rigor: Severe shaking chill.

Ringing in the ears: Medically called tinnitus, this can arise in any of "the four sections of the ear" -- the outer ear, the middle ear, the inner ear, and the brain -- and can be due to many causes including ear infections, fluid in the ears, Meniere syndrome (the combination of tinnitus and deafness), some medications such as aspirin and other nonsteroidal antiinflammatory drugs (NSAIDs), aging, and ear trauma (such as from the noise of planes, firearms, or loud music).

Risk Analysis: Generally, the science of risks, their probability and evaluation. In business, it is a technique to identify and assess factors that may jeopardize the success of a project or achieving a goal. This technique also helps to define preventive measures to reduce the probability of these factors from occurring and identify countermeasures to successfully deal with these constraints when they develop to avert possible negative effects on the competitiveness of the company.

Risk Mitigation: Long-term measures for reducing or eliminating risk.

Risk: A form of uncertainty that has a well-grounded (quantitative) probability. Risk = (probability of something happening) x (consequences if it does happen).

Risorius.(L. risor, laughter). Pertaining to a facial muscle, i.e., musculus risorius.

S

Salpingo-(G. salpinx, trumpet). Pertaining to a muscle fascicle attached to the eustachian (auditory) tube and pharynx.

Saphenous.(G. saphenes, visible) Pertaining to a muscle that is associated with the saphenous vein.

Sarcolemma. Plasma membrane of a muscle cell

Sarcomere. Functional unit in a muscle cell; Z line to Z line

Sarcoplasm. Cytoplasm of a muscle cell

Sarcoplasmic reticulum. The endoplasmic reticulum in a muscle cell

Satellite cells. Cells found in skeletal muscle which are dormant stem cells

Scala tympani. Chamber within the the cochlear duct

Scala vestibule. Chamber within the the cochlear duct

Schlemm's canal. Circular canal near the junction of the cornea and

Sartorius.(L. sartor, a tailor). Musculus sartorius.

Scabrous. Roughly and irregularly rugose.

Scape. The first, elongate segment of the antenna next to the head.

Sclerite. A general term for any single plate of the exoskeleton.

Scrobe. Large groove for the reception of an appendage, such as the antennal scrobe.

Segment. A joint.

Serrate. With teeth along the edge, saw-like.

Seta (plural: setae). Hair.

Shagreened. With a fine and close set roughness, such as shark skin.

Spiracle. An orifice of the tracheal system where gases enter and leave the body. Ants have 9 or 10 spiracles on each side of the body.

Spongiform tissue or process. Specialized sponge-like external cuticular tissue found mainly on the waist segments in some groups of ants.

Spur. Spine-like appendage, may be paired or pectinate, and found at the end of the tibia.

Squamate. Scale-shaped.

Sternal. Pertaining to the sternum or lower portion of the body.

Sternite. The lower sclerite of a segment.

Sting. The modified ovipositer found on female ants at the apex of the gaster, sharp and often ejecting a venomous secretion.

Stria (plural: striae). A fine, impressed line, usually longitudinal in orientation.

Striate. With striae or multiple impressed hairs.

Striate-punctate. Rows of punctures.

Striga (plural: strigae). A narrow, transverse line.

Strigate. Transversely striate.

Subdecumbent. Referring to a hair standing approximately 45 degrees from the body surface.

Suberect. Referring to a hair bending approximately 10 to 20 degrees from vertical.

Subpetiolar process. An anteroventral projection on the petiole or its peduncle, may be absent.

Sulcate. Being deeply furrowed or grooved.

Sulcus. Deep furrow or groove.

Suture. Seam or line that separates two body plates.

Scalenus.(G. skalenos, uneven). Pertaining to muscles having uneven sides or length.

Scapulo-(L. scapulae, shoulder blades). Pertaining to a muscle associated with the scapula.

Schizogony: Asexual reproductive stage of malaria parasites. In red blood cells, schizogony entails development of a single trophozoite into numerous merozoites. A similar process happens in infected liver cells.

Schizont: A developmental form of the malaria parasite that contains many merozoites. Schizonts are seen in the liver-stage and blood-stage parasites.

sclera which allows the aqueous humor to drain from the anterior chamber

Schmidt-Lanterman cleft.Cytoplasm of a Schwann cell

Schwann cells.Cells which form the myelin sheath in the peripheral nervous system

Sebaceous gland. Gland which produces and secrete sebum

Sebum. Oily secretion

Secondary follicle. Antral follicle; follicle after the fluid filled antrum forms

Seminiferous tubules. Tubules where spermatozoa mature

Septal cell. Type II alveolar cell

Serosa. Lining of closed body cavities

Serous cell. Cell which secretes watery secretion containing enzymes

Serous demilune. Serous cell which is a moon shaped cap resting on a mucous secreting cell in a salivary gland

Sertoli cells. Supporting cells in the testes

Sharpey's fibers. Collagen fibers in bone; peforating fibers

Simple epithelium. Epithelium consisting of a single layer of cells

Simple gland.A gland with an unbranched duct or no duct

Sinusoid. Wide, leaky capillary

Slit pore. Opening between the foot processes of podocytes in the kidney

Small alveolar cell. Type I alveolar cell

Small granule cell. Argyrophilic cell or dense core granule cell

Smoth endoplasmic reticulum. Endoplasmic reticulum that is not studded with ribosomes

Smudge cell.A fragmented white blood which became fragmented while making the peripheral blood smear slide

Smooth muscle.involuntary muscle which does not have cross striations

Soma. Cell body of a neuron

Somatotroph. Cell type found in the adenohypophysis which secretes growth hormone

Space of Disse. Perisinuoidal space seen in the liver

Space of Mall. Space seen in the liver at the periphery of a portal canal

Spermatid. Spermatogenic cell

Spermatocyte. Spermatogenic cell

Spermatogonia. Spermatogenic cell

Spermatozoa. Mature sperm cell

Spicules. Trabeculae seen in spongy bone

Splenic cords. Cords of Billroth; tissue between the splenic sinuses

Spongy bone. Cancellous bone; trabecular bone

Squamocolumnar junction. Transition region between the exocervix and endocervix where the epithelium changes from stratified squamous to simple columnar

Squamous. Flat

Squamous epithelium. Epithelium where the surface cells are flat; can be either simple or stratified

Stab. Immature neutrophil in which the nucleus is not yet multi-lobed; also called a band cell

Stellate. Shaped like a star

Stem cell. Undifferentiate precursor cell

Stereocilia. Very long microvilli found on some epithelial cells

Stratified epithelium. Epithelium composed of more than one layer of cells

Stratum. Layer

Stratum basale.1. Basal layer of the epidermis; also called the stratum germinativum2. Basal layer of the endometrium

Stratum corneum. Most external layer of the epidermis; also called the horny layer

Stratum functionalis. Portion of the endometrium which is shed monthly

Stratum germinativum. Basal layer of the epidermis; also called stratum basale

Semi-(L. semis, half). Prefix denoting half or partly.

Sensitivity: 1. In psychology, the quality of being sensitive. As, for example, sensitivity training, training in small groups to develop a sensitive awareness and understanding of oneself and of ones relationships with others. 2. In disease epidemiology, the ability of a system to detect epidemics and other changes in disease occurrence. 3. In screening for a disease, the proportion of persons with the disease who are correctly identified by a screening test. 4. In the definition of a disease, the proportion of persons with the disease who are correctly identified by defined criteria.

Sequelae: Morbid conditions following as a consequence of a disease.

Serology: The branch of science dealing with the measurement and characterization of antibodies and other immunological substances in body fluids, particularly serum.

Serratus.(L. serra, saw). Pertaining to muscles that are serrated, notched, or dentate.

Shortness of breath: Difficulty in breathing. Medically referred to as dyspnea. Shortness of breath can be caused by respiratory (breathing passages and lungs) or circulatory (heart and blood vessels) conditions. See also dyspnea.

Soleus.(L. solea, a sandal [foot]). Musculus soleus.

Sore throat: Pain in the throat. Sore throat may be caused by many different causes, including inflammation of the larynx, pharynx, or tonsils.

Sore: 1. (adjective) A popular term for painful. I have sore fingers from typing dictionary terms. She has a sore throat. 2. (noun) A nondescript term for nearly any lesion of the skin or mucous membranes. He has a number of sores in his mouth.

Species: Organisms in the same genus that have similar characteristics.

Spinous.(L. spina, thorn). Related to the spinous processes of the vertebral column.

Splenectomy: Removal of the spleen.

Splenius.(G. splenion, a bandage). Musculus splenius and others.

Splenomegaly: Enlargement of the spleen. Found in some malaria patients. Splenomegaly can be used to measure malaria endemicity during surveys (e.g., in communities or in schoolchildren).

Sporozoite rate: The proportion of female anopheline mosquitoes of a particular species that have sporozoites in their salivary glands (as seen by dissection), or that are positive in immunologic tests to detect sporozoite antigens.

Sporozoite: A stage in the life cycle of the malaria parasite. Sporozoites are produced in the mosquito and migrate to the mosquito's salivary glands.

Stapedius.(L. stapes, stirrup). A muscle inserted into the stapes. Musculus stapedius.

Sterno-(G. sternon, the chest). Pertaining to muscles attached to the sternum.

Stomach: The digestive organ that is located in the upper abdomen, under the ribs. The upper part of the stomach connects to the esophagus, and the lower part leads into the small intestine.

Strain: A genetic variant within a species.

Stratum granulosum. Granular layer of the epidermis

Stratum lucidum. Clear layer of the epidermis; found only in thick skin

Stratum spinosum. Spiny layer of the epidermis

Stratum vasculare. Central layer in myometrium

Striated border. Visible effect of the microvilli in the small intestine; also called the brush border

Striated duct. Duct with infoldings of plasma membrane and mitochondria as to give it a striped appearance

Stria vascularis. Part of the wall of the cochlear duct

Striated muscle. Skeletal muscle and cardiac muscle

Stroma. The supporting tissue in an organ, i.e the blood vessels, connective tissue, nerves, etc.

Subcapsular sinus. Space underneath a lymph node capsule

Submucosa. Tissue layer underneath the mucosa

Stylo-(G. stylos, pillar or post). Pertaining to muscles attached to the styloid process of the temporal bone.

Sub-(L. sub, under). Denoting muscles that are beneath or inferior to a named structure, e.g., subclavius.

Subneural clefts. Folds or gutters in the sarcolemma

Substantia propria. Layers of collagen which form the cornea

Sudoriferous glands. Sweat gland

Sustentacular cell. Supporting cell

Synapse. Cell junction between neurons

Syncytium. Mass formed by cells which have merged with each other

Sulfadoxine-pyrimethamine: A drug used against malaria. Its value has been compromised by the emergence of drug-resistant malaria parasites

Sunscreen: A substance that blocks the effect of the sun's harmful rays. Using lotions that contain sunscreens can reduce the risk of skin cancer, including melanoma.

Superior.(L. superus, above). Denoting a muscle located above another muscle in an inferior position or to another structure to which it is attached.

Supinator.(L. supinare, to place on back). Denoting a muscle that, upon contraction, rotates the forearm and hand with the palm facing anteriorly when the hand and forearm are in the anatomical position.

Suppressive treatment: Treatment intended to prevent clinical symptoms and parasitemia through destruction of parasites in red blood cells.

Supra-(L. supra, above). Prefix to note the position of a muscle above a named structure, e.g., supracostalis.

Suralis.(L. sura, calf of the leg). Relating to the calf.

Surgery: The branch of medicine that employs operations in the treatment of disease or injury. Surgery can involve cutting, abrading, suturing, or otherwise physically changing body tissues and organs.

Sweating: The act of secreting fluid from the skin by the sweat (sudoriferous) glands. These are small tubular glands situated within and under the skin (in the subcutaneous tissue). They discharge by tiny openings in the surface of the skin.

T

T cell. Type of lymphocyte which is involved in cellular immunity

T tubule. Invagination of the plasma membrane seen in muscle fibers which allows for rapid calcium distribution

Taste buds. Structures found on some papillae in the tongue and in mucous membrane of the pharynx

Taste pore. Opening in the taste bud

Tectorial membrane. Membrane within the cochlea of the inner ear

Tendon organ. Encapsulated nerve endings stimulated by stretching

Tenia coli. Modification of the muscularis externa of the large intestine

Terminal bouton. Rounded flask like region at the end of a neuron

Terminal bronchioles. Bronchioles just before the respiratory branch

Theca externa. Layer of connective tissue on the outer portion of the follicle;

outside the theca interna

Theca folliculi. Layer of cells around a primary follicle in the ovary

Theca interna. Layer of tissue underneath the theca externa

Theca lutein cells. Peripherally located in the corpus luteum

Thick filaments. Myosin filaments

Thin filaments. Actin filaments

Thromoboctye. Platelet

Thyroid follicle. Spherical collection of thyroid cells which surrounds colloid

Thyrotrop. Cell type in the anterior pituitary which secretes TSH

Tight junctions.Type of junction between epithelial cells

Tissue.A group of cells working together to perform a similar function. The four primary tissue types are: epithelial, connective, muscular, nervous

Tonofilament. Type of protein filament

Totipotential cell. Cell that is able to develop into a variety of different cell types; undifferentiated cell

Trabeculae. Spicules

Trabecular bone. Spongy bone; cancellous bone

Transitional epithelium. Type of epithelium found in the urinary tract

Transverse tubule. Invagination of the plasma membrane seen in muscle fibers which allows for rapid calcium distribution; T tubule

Trophoblast. Outer layer on the blastocyst

Tubular gland. Gland where the secretory part is tubular

Tubuli recti. Small channels lined by sertoli cells in the testis; straight tubules

Tubuloalveolar gland. Tubular gland which has a saclike portion at the end of the tube

Tunica adventitia. Outer layer of a blood vessel which is composed primarily of connective tissue

Tunica albuginea. Tough connective tissue covering a structure

Tunica intima. Innermost layer of a blood vessel or other tubular structure

Tunica media. Middle layer of vessels composed of smooth muscle

Tunica vaginalis. Membrane around the testis

Type II alveolar cell.Cell of the pulmonary alveoli which secretes surfactant

Temporalis.(L. tempus, time or temple). Relating to the temple, musculus temporalis.

Tachycardia: Increased heart rate.

Tachypnea: Increased rate of breathing.

Tarsus. A collective term for the five apical segments of any leg.

Tergal. Dorsal.

Tergite. The upper sclerite of a segment.

Thorax. The second major body section, which consists of three body sections: pro-, meso-, and metathorax) In ants and other hymenopterans, the thorax is fused with the first segment of the abdomen, the propodeum. The combined thorax and propodeum form the alitrunk.

Tibia. (plural: tibiae). The fourth segment of the leg found between the femur and the tarsus.

Torulus. The small annular sclerite that surrounds the antennal socket.

Trochanter. The short second segment of the leg, just following the coxa and preceding the femur.

Tubercle. A small, rounded protuberance.

Tubercle. Covered with tubercles (small thick spines).

Tensor.(L. tendere, to stretch). Pertaining to a muscle whose function is to make a structure, to which it is attached, firm and tense.

Teres.(L. tero, round or smooth). Denoting certain muscles that are round and long.

Tetracycline: An antibiotic drug that can be used against malaria for treatment only, not prevention.

Throat: The throat is the anterior (front) portion of the neck beginning at the back of the mouth, consisting anatomically of the pharynx and **larynx.** The throat contains the trachea and a portion of the esophagus.

Thrombocytopenia: Low platelet count that can lead to impaired blood clotting and spontaneous bleeding.

Thyro-(G. thyreos, an oblong shield). Denoting certain muscles attached to the thyroid cartilage.

Tibialis.(L. tibia, a pipe or flute). Pertaining to muscles attached to the tibia.

Tinnitus: Ringing sound in the ears, a common side effect of quinine treatment.

Tiredness: See: Tired.

Trachelian.(G. trachelos, neck). Pertaining to muscles associated with the neck.

Transactional Environment: Factors which are external to an organisation as such, but which the organisation may be able to influence (e.g. through information campaigns, legal actions, lobbying, etc.).

Transversus.(L. trans, across + vertare, to turn). Denoting muscles that lie across the long axis of an organ or a part.

Trapezius.(G. trapezion, a table) A four sided muscle having no two sides that are parallel. Musculus trapezius.

Triangularis.(L. tri, three + angulus, angle). A muscle that is, more or less, triangular in shape.

Triceps.(L. tri, three + caput, head). Denoting a muscle with three heads, e.g., musculus triceps.

Triticeo-(L. triticum, a grain of wheat). Pertaining to a muscle attached in part to the cartilago triticea.

Trophozoite: A developmental form during the blood stage of malaria parasites. After merozoites have invaded the red blood cell, they develop into trophozoites (sometimes, early trophozoites are called "rings" or "ring stage parasites"); trophozoites develop into schizonts.

U

Uncertainty (Genuine Uncertainty): While risk is a form of uncertainty that has a well-grounded (quantitative) probability, genuine uncertainty cannot be ascribed a probability.

Uncinatus.(L. uncus, hook). Os hamatum or unciform bone. A muscle attached to the hook of the hamate, e.g., pisiuncinatus.

Unilocular adipose tissue. White adipose tissue; adult adipose tissue

Unipolar neuron. Neuron with one process which immediately divides; pseudounipolar neuron

Urinary space. Space between the glomerular capillaries and Bowman's capsule

Uriniferous tubule.A component of the nephron

Utricle. One of the sacs in the inner ear

Uvea. Vascular tunic of the eye

Ulnaris.(L. ulna, elbow forearm). Pertaining to the larger and more medial of the two bones of the forearm.

Urethrae.(G. ourethra, urethra). Relating to the urethra, e. g., musculus sphincter urethrae.

Urine: Liquid waste produced by the kidneys. Urine is a clear, transparent fluid that normally has an amber color.

V

Vaccine: A preparation that stimulates an immune response that can prevent an infection or create resistance to an infection.

Vacuole. An apparently empty space within a cell

Valve of Kerckring. Plica circulares

Varicose vein. Twisted, dilated vein

Vasa nervorum. Blood vessels which supply a nerve trunk

Vasa recta. Blood vessels which form a hairpin-like loop within the kidney

Venous portal system. Vein which is between two capillary beds; an example is the hepatic portal systme

Venous sinus. Large channel for venous blood

Ventricular fold. Fold of the mucous membrane in the larynx

Venule. Small vein

Vestibular membrane. Membrane within the cochlea which separates the scala media from the scala vestibuli

Villi. Fingerlike projections seen on the mucosa of the small intestine

Volkmann's canals. Channels in compact bone which run transversely

Von Ebner's glands. Serous glands associated with circumvallate papilla

Vaginae.(L. vagina, sheath). Pertaining to a muscle attached to a joint capsule.

Variable: A quantity or quality capable of assuming a set of values or conditions.

Vastus.(L. vastus, huge). A large muscle of the thigh, musculus quadriceps with three vasti and a rectus.

Vector competence: The ability of a vector (e.g., *Anopheles* mosquitoes) to transmit a disease (e.g., malaria).

Vector: An organism (e.g., *Anopheles* mosquitoes) that transmits an infectious agent (e.g. malaria parasites) from one host to the other (e.g., humans).

Venter. The lower surface.

Ventral. The lower surface.

Verrucose. With irregularly shaped lobes or wart-like protuberances.

Vertex. Upper surface of head between eyes, frons, and occiput.

Virus: A microorganism composed of a piece of genetic material - RNA or DNA - surrounded by a protein coat. To replicate, a virus must infect a cell and direct its cellular machinery to produce new viruses.

Vivax: See *Plasmodium*

W

Wharton's jelly. Mucous connective tissue found in the umbilical cord

White blood cells. Leukocytes

White fibers. Type of muscle fibers which make up fast-twitch motor units

White matter. Region of the central nervous system with abundant myelination and no cell bodies

White pulp. Lymphatic tissue of the spleen

Whole mount. Slide preparation technique using the whole specimen

Woven bone. Immature bone; non-lamelllar bone

Waist. The isolated body segments between the alitrunk and the gaster, sometimes called the pedicel, but waist is the preferred term.

X

Xenia – the effect of pollen on seeds and fruit

Xeromorphic leaves. Leaves with special structural adaptations to living in a dry environment.

Xerophyte. A plant adapted to growth and survival in a dry environment.

Xylem elements. Cells comprising the xylem.

Xylem ray. That portion of a vascular ray which is found in the xylem.

Xylem. Water conducting tissue containing tracheary elements.

Xylotomy. The anatomical study of wood.

Y

Yellow marrow. Bone marrow consisting primarily of adipose cells

Z

Zoonosis: A disease that naturally occurs in animals that can also occur in humans.

Zoophilic: Zoophilic mosquitoes are mosquitoes that prefer to take blood meals on animals. Z disc/Z line.Dark line in the center of the I band; Z line to Z line defines a sarcomere

Chloroquine and Body Tissues

Zona fasciculate. The middle layer of the adrenal cortex; produces glucocorticoids

Zona glomerulosa. The outer layer of the adrenal cortex where mineralocorticoids are produced

Zona pellucid. Glycoprotein coat around the oocyte

Zona reticularis. Innermost layer of the adrenal cortex; produces sex steroids

Zonula adherens. Type of junction between epithelial cells; intermediate junction

Zonula occludens. Type of junction between epithelial cells; tight junction

Zonular fibers. Suspensory ligament of the lens

Zygote. Diploid cell; fertilized ovum

Zymogenic cells. Chief cells; cells which secrete enzymes

Zygomaticus.(G. zygoma, a bar or bolt) Pertaining to the zygomatic bone, e.g., musculus zygomaticus.

Chloroquine and Body Tissues